Wisdom
OF THE
Plant Devas

"What a fitting title for a marvelous book! From the opening paragraph when Thea enticingly invites us into the magical realm of the plant devas to the ending story about uva ursi, I was thoroughly and completely captivated. Though I've experienced this sacred relationship with the plants and have read about it in several other excellent books, Thea's account is refreshingly unique, deeply authentic, and easily accessible to the reader. She makes what at times may seem unbelievable to some—the ability to converse with other life-forms—to be fully believable and accessible to anyone. Woven into *Wisdom of the Plant Devas* is Thea's own wonderful story and heartfelt deep relationship with plant devas. My only criticism is that I was sorry when the book ended. I wanted more!"

ROSEMARY GLADSTAR,
HERBALIST AND FOUNDER OF UNITED PLANT SAVERS,
AUTHOR OF *ROSEMARY GLADSTAR'S FAMILY HERBAL* AND
PLANTING THE FUTURE

"The plants continue to turn up the volume urging us to listen to their guidance for our spiritual evolution. *Wisdom of the Plant Devas* is the next level of communication with the green beings, revealing important information not only about our personal growth and planetary transformation but also about our connection to the entire universe. Thea Summer Deer shares her communication with the plant devas, the architects who help deepen our relationship to the spirit of the plant, with amazing clarity, love, and light. This book is a must read for all people wanting to take up their rightful relational place in the vast web of life both earthly and beyond."

PAM MONTGOMERY,
AUTHOR OF *PLANT SPIRIT HEALING*

"The devas will tell you their stories, recite their poetry, regale you with pronouncements, and show you their portraits. You may fall in love. You may never return."

SUSUN S. WEED,
AUTHOR OF *WISE WOMAN HERBAL SERIES*

"Bravo! This is my new favorite plant book! To take it a step further, it is one I wish I had written. *Wisdom of the Plant Devas* is a rich and generous treasure trove of information and inspiration and an articulate expression of the power of spirit in medicine."

NICKI SCULLY,
AUTHOR OF *PLANETARY HEALING: SPIRIT MEDICINE FOR GLOBAL TRANSFORMATION* AND *POWER ANIMAL MEDITATIONS*

"In this lovely book, Thea Summer Deer takes us on a fascinating journey into the hidden world of the plant devas and shares their powerful message of Earth wisdom, transformation, and healing."

NATHANIEL ALTMAN,
AUTHOR OF *THE DEVA HANDBOOK* AND *THE HONEY PRESCRIPTION*

Wisdom
OF THE
Plant Devas

HERBAL MEDICINE
FOR A NEW EARTH

Thea Summer Deer

Bear & Company
Rochester, Vermont • Toronto, Canada

Bear & Company
One Park Street
Rochester, Vermont 05767
www.BearandCompanyBooks.com

Bear & Company is a division of Inner Traditions International

Copyright © 2011 by Cynthia L. Stacey

All rights reserved. No part of this book may be reproduced or utilized in any form or by any means, electronic or mechanical, including photocopying, recording, or by any information storage and retrieval system, without permission in writing from the publisher.

Note to the reader: *This book is intended as an informational guide. The remedies, approaches, and techniques described herein are meant to supplement, and not to be a substitute for, professional medical care or treatment. They should not be used to treat a serious ailment without prior consultation with a qualified health care professional.*

Library of Congress Cataloging-in-Publication Data
Deer, Thea Summer.
  Wisdom of the plant Devas : herbal medicine for a new earth / Thea Summer Deer.
      p. cm.
  Includes bibliographical references and index.
  ISBN 978-1-59143-085-8 (pbk.) — 978-1-59143-941-7 (ebook)
  1. Materia medica, Vegetable. 2. Medicinal plants. 3. Herbs—Therapeutic use. I. Title.
  RS164.D353 2011
  615.3'21—dc23

                                                                    2011023504

Printed and bound in the United States by Versa Press

10   9   8   7   6   5   4   3   2   1

Text design and layout by Virginia Scott Bowman
This book was typeset in Garamond Premier Pro and Myriad Pro

Illustration concept and design by Thea Summer Deer
Botanical and digital illustrations by Adam Bruce Caddick
Photography by Marion Z. Skydancer with additional photography by Thea Summer Deer
Digital manipulation by Adam Bruce Caddick, Marion Z. Skydancer, and Thea Summer Deer

To send correspondence to the author of this book, mail a first-class letter to the author c/o Inner Traditions • Bear & Company, One Park Street, Rochester, VT 05767, and we will forward the communication.

This book is dedicated foremost to my mother, Alice Jean Stacey, in whose garden my childhood imagination ran wild, and to my father, George Lewis Stacey, who watched me run wild and admired my courage. Without your nurturing and support the following book would not have been possible. And to all my children—natural born, not-yet-born, adopted, step-parented, or otherwise loved, and to their children's children's children—it is my greatest wish that yours be a legacy of light, because your elders were willing to embrace their darkness.

"The Invocation to Kali, Part 5," © 1971 by May Sarton, from *Collected Poems 1930–1993* by May Sarton. Used by permission of W. W. Norton & Company, Inc.

"The Tao is called the Great Mother/. . . ." from *Tao Te Ching by Lao Tzu, A New English Version*, with foreword and notes by Stephen Mitchell. Translation © 1988 by Stephen Mitchell. Reprinted by permission of HarperCollins Publishers.

"Out Beyond Ideas" from *The Essential Rumi* by Jalal al-Din Muhammad Rumi, translated by Coleman Barks, © 1995 by Coleman Barks, reproduced with permission.

"The Song of the Self Heal Fairy" from *The Complete Book of the Flower Fairies* by Cicely Mary Barker, © 2002 by the estate of Cicely Mary Barker, reproduced with permission of the Penguin Group, Inc.

"Weeds" by Phillip Pulfrey, *Perspectives*, © 2010 by Phillip Pulfrey, reproduced with permission.

Lyrics from the songs "Let Us Ride" and "Rainbow Song" by Sananda Ra, © 2006 by Sananda Ra, reproduced with permission.

Lyrics from the song "New Ground Breaking" by Charles E. Willhide, © 1995 by Charles E. Willhide, reproduced with permission

Lyrics from the song "6 Winds" by John M. Roman, © 2006 by John M. Roman, reproduced with permission.

Help us to be the always hopeful
Gardeners of the spirit
Who know that without darkness
Nothing comes to birth
As without light
Nothing flowers.

MAY SARTON

Contents

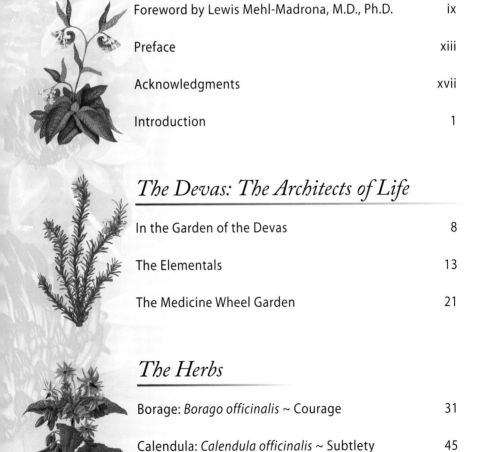

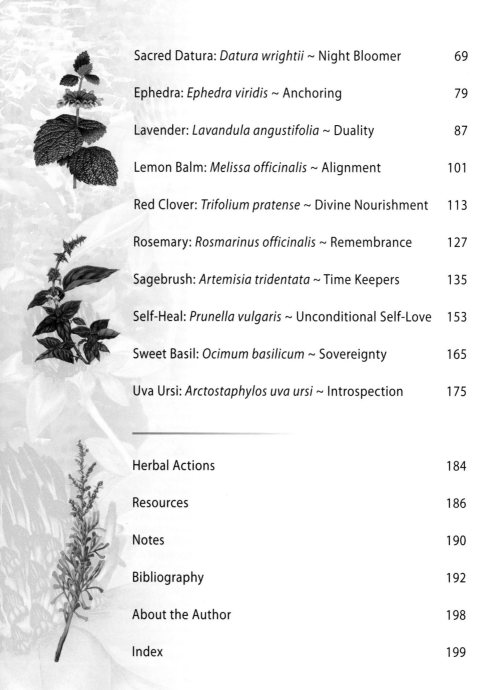

Foreword

Wisdom of the Plant Devas: Herbal Medicine for a New Earth is timely and needed, especially in the way that Thea approaches it, as a guide to connecting with the herbs and the spirits of the devas through their stories. My own work has been about the healing power of ceremony and story. In *Coyote Medicine,* I wrote about my evolution through conventional medicine to come to study Native American healing; in *Coyote Healing,* I wrote about the ceremonies and rituals associated with so-called miraculous cures; and in *Coyote Wisdom,* I wrote about the stories and their power to inspire healing. The stories the devas tell through Thea are just such stories. These stories inspire us to greet the herbs and their spirits, to recognize them in a deep and profound manner, and to carry the herbs into our lives in the same way that people carry the stories of healers with them for years, letting them work their magic over time. *Wisdom of the Plant Devas* can work similar magic as we carry their stories with us, contemplating their power and wisdom, letting them do their magic of healing on us.

My own children are named for herbs, perhaps to their chagrin. First came Redwood Sorrel (Sorrel for short) and then Yarrow. I suppose this perpetually marks them as children from the Birkenstock and granola era of the '70s, but those were also times of dramatic renewal of our relationship with nature and the plant kingdom, as evidenced in the birth of publications like *Magic of Findhorn* and *Mother Earth News.* The names Sorrel and Yarrow reflected my fascination with herbs and honored my Cherokee ancestors' tradition of naming children after nature. I have always been intrigued by the idea of communicating with the spirits of the plants and have used herbs in my work in the medicine ways since the 1970s. I regularly bring sweetgrass, sage, basil, and lavender to ceremony and have a great affinity with the spirits of these plants. These spirits support the healing work that I do with people and have served me well.

The premise of *Wisdom of the Plant Devas* is that you can call on the spirits of the herbs for healing even if you are not in their presence. This takes the herbs to another level, that of their spiritual ability to help guide and heal without being physically present. Thea also likes tinctures, teas, and infusions, but this book creates a bridge between the botanical medical use of herbs and the spirit medicine use. In our learning about the connectedness of All That Is, we transcend the barriers of time and space to call on any herb to be present with us and assist in our growth and our healing. In my work of bridging the worlds of allopathic medicine and traditional Native medicine, I find these ideas very supportive, including the insistence that using a plant is invoking its spirit and that we need to honor that spirit even as we use the physical plant. Thea's contribution is to inspire us to create a new dialogue between the seen and unseen worlds and ourselves. By working with *Wisdom of the Plant Devas*, Thea points out that we can use the spiritual essence of the plant wherever we are, even if we are unable to find the physical herb itself.

Writing this book took deep listening on Thea's part, listening to the voices of the herbs themselves and communicating that essence with us. She developed these deep listening skills by spending large amounts of time in nature and by listening to the inner voice that writes her songs. I have known Thea as a mother, a midwife, a musician, and a fellow journeyer on the medicine path. We worked together with Resources for World Health, a nonprofit organization whose aim was to support medicine people and ceremonies around North America. We participated in ceremony throughout the United States and even abroad in Europe. I have seen Thea draw on her higher wisdom and guidance in all these contexts, and it is exciting to see her apply this to the spirits of the herbs.

Thea's work will be helpful to me in organizing my own thoughts about the various plant spirits. It will also increase others' awareness of how close the plants are to us. It will help people to appreciate the energetics of the herbs, to realize that the plant kingdom is not lower on the hierarchy of evolution, and to become aware that, in some ways, they are more evolved than people are. They so quickly adapt to changing conditions, a timely lesson for all of us. We would do well to increase our awareness of the intelligence that exists in nature. It is our sense of superiority and lack of awareness of our dependence on nature for our survival that threaten the continued existence of our species. The devas hold all the genetic memory of a plant, even once something has become extinct, and they can potentially bring it back from extinction if it is determined that the need is great and that it will assist us in our spiritual evolution. They are just beginning to show us how powerful they are as aids in our evolution. Never have we had a greater need.

LEWIS MEHL-MADRONA

Lewis Mehl-Madrona, M.D., Ph.D., is certified in family practice, geriatrics, and psychiatry and holds a Ph.D. in clinical psychology. He worked for years in rural emergency medicine and is currently a core faculty member in the clinical psychology program at Union Institute and University in Brattleboro, Vermont. He is the author of *Coyote Healing, Coyote Wisdom,* and the bestselling *Coyote Medicine.* His latest books are *Narrative Medicine: The Use of History and Story in the Healing Process* and *Healing the Mind through the Power of Story: The Promise of Narrative Psychiatry.*

New Ground Breaking

Cowering through life, just to survive.
Never pulling my head from the sand.
Only talking 'bout how to become alive.
But never really finding who I am.

Answers to mysteries seem too much to bear.
I'm not even sure of the questions.
Sometimes it's too much to even care.
It's hard to see life's suggestions. But

I can find that peace of mind,
already here for the taking.
Now it's time to see the sign.
I feel new ground is breaking.

Calmness seems like the distant moon.
Always there but never reaching.
But it feels good just to stay in tune.
Listening for all life is teaching, and . . .

Souls search for truer ways.
Always looking for better days.
Working to find out what's in me.
When all I have to do is . . . let it be.

So if you feel like you've come undone,
listen for what life is showing.
And connect yourself to the rising sun.
It will carry you to knowing.

CHARLES E. WILLHIDE

Preface

*Watching gardeners label their plants, I vow with all beings
to practice the old horticulture and let the plants identify me.*

ROBERT AIKEN

Light filtered through the kitchen window and onto the kitchen counter
where I was working one bright, crisp morning in my Carolina mountain
home. Cooking is one of my passions, and I was developing a new recipe. As
I stood in the kitchen in front of the spice rack, looking for just the right
hint of spice for my latest epicurean adventure, opening jars and smelling my
way through the homegrown herbs, rosemary practically leapt off the shelf
and into my hand. I removed the lid and with eyes closed deeply inhaled her
warm and piney scent. "Perfect," I thought. And then I heard a voice: "If rosemary has appeared in your cards today . . ." It dawned on me in that moment
that I might be experiencing something similar to divining with herbs. I was
intuitively "pulling" the right herbs off the shelf as one might pull a card
from an oracle deck. These herbs were literally talking to me! And so began
Wisdom of the Plant Devas: Herbal Medicine for a New Earth. The messages
that came through were ones that the devas had obviously been waiting to
share. The copious writing that followed and the ensuing revelations became
a catalyst for personal growth and change.

While I first heard the voice of an herb deva in my kitchen that morning,
shortly thereafter, they appeared in my garden. Nearing the end of my fertile

years and incredibly grateful for my partner and our committed relationship, I felt the impulse to offer some of the last of my menstrual blood, mixed with his semen, to a wild black raspberry bush that grew in our backyard next to the vegetable garden. My partner was receptive to the idea, but then he isn't called the GreenMan for nothing! It had been my intention to give something sacred to me, to us, back to the earth. The devas were ecstatic. I had to rub my eyes in disbelief. These little luminous beings were jumping up and down with joy and were delighted that I had made this secret offering. (So much for secrets!) Then they sent me off running to my computer, so I could type the messages they were so insistent on delivering. Later, upon reading what I had written, I was astounded. I had no idea that such a simple act would bring such a powerful vision. They show up frequently now, when I am working in my garden, and more often than not I have to put everything aside and go promptly to my computer to deliver their timely message.

My fascination with herbs and medicinal plants began early, when I started gathering them in the mountains of North Carolina, where I spent my childhood summers. I have always counted my blessings and know that I am very fortunate to have spent a great deal of time in nature. My parents raised me in a traditional Seminole Indian village, and it was there that I ran barefoot, rode my pony, climbed coconut trees, and fished along the banks of the Miami River. When I was eight, we moved to the rural countryside, where I rode horses through mango, avocado, and lime groves; swam in the ocean; and played in my mother's award-winning rose garden. My mother regularly took me to visit other amazing gardens as well, including the Fairchild Tropical Botanic Garden and the Vizcaya Museum and Gardens in South Miami, Florida, and the Butchart Gardens in Victoria, British Columbia, Canada. I think these places soothed her soul, and when the soul of the mother is soothed, the child knows herself to be in a safe place.

My sister left home when I was less than a year old, so I practically grew up as an only child. Like most children who spend a lot of time alone, I developed imaginary playmates, some of which were nature spirits that appeared in various luminous forms. Fairy rings emerged frequently in the acreage behind my house, where the horses grazed and the wild bunnies invited me into their dens to meet their adorable little babies. I have a very fertile and active imagination. I also have the natural gift of clairvoyance and clairaudience, which facilitated my ability to contact the realms of spirit, particularly the spirits of the plants of which I write.

In my late teens I lived and worked at a plant nursery in South Florida that specialized in orchids, bromeliads, and cacti. I loved these plants and spent hours observing and drawing them. In my twenties I grew herbs like comfrey and red raspberry for use in my midwifery practice, with great success. Over time I developed a kinesthetic relationship with the herbs, sensing their subtle energies and responding to their demands for inclusion in various culinary creations or medicinal preparations. They had been waiting to share their wisdom with me once I learned how to listen. My practical knowledge of their healing abilities, or even my experience in taste and food combining, took me only so far. The devas of the herbs, however, were challenging me to explore beyond my realm of knowledge and experience. They emphasized that our food *is* our medicine, and not only for our physical body but also for our spiritual body. Herbs are some of the most powerful allies we have for these times.

As a young woman I wasn't content just playing with herbs in my kitchen and garden, and became serious about pursuing my studies. I became a midwife and one of the founding mothers of the South Florida School of Midwifery. As executive director of Resources for World Health, I worked with indigenous healers from all over the world. Then I pursued a course of study at the BotanoLogos School for Herbal Studies. While my background is firmly rooted in the European herbal tradition, BotanoLogos opened my mind to the world of medical herbalism and Chinese five element theory.

Neither did I neglect my spiritual studies during this time. I pursued my interest in the magical realms by becoming a student of occult mysticism in my teens, a devotee of an East Indian guru in my twenties, and a seeker of shamanism in my thirties. During my thirties and forties I helped support myself as a singer-songwriter playing in bars, coffeehouses, and restaurants. I had been playing guitar since I was eight, and I write a lot of songs about mountains, rivers, and canyons. This love of nature and music has facilitated my ability to tune in to the voices of the devas. There is always a song to be found in nature, and I am always listening for it.

Today, I have come full circle. Presently in my fifties, I achieve inner peace by tending to my garden, playing my guitar, and spending time with my granddaughters. I live in the Appalachian Mountains of my childhood, surrounded by Cherokee ancestral land. It was here that I learned how to shoot a bow, canoe, weave, and gather medicinal herbs. These mountains are some of the oldest in the world, and they boast the widest variety of herbs anywhere on Earth.

While this book discusses only the smallest handful of herbs, it is meant to provide a blueprint through which to view the world of nature, healing, and transformation. Choosing which herbs to write about was an impossible task, so I gave it up to the devas and let the plants choose me. These are simply the ones that showed up.

Wisdom of the Plant Devas: Herbal Medicine for a New Earth is intended to be a spiritual guide, and while it contains factual information about herbs, it is not meant to be a garden guide or a resource for plant identification. Nor is it meant for diagnosing or as a how-to for making herbal recommendations or preparations. Rather, my intention was to take the best of what has come before, the sum of what we know—or think we know—about an herb, and use that information as a springboard to attain an enlightened understanding of how that plant can now serve us. When we make a direct connection with an herb and allow it to directly inform us, we become less dependent on looking outside of ourselves and to the experts for advice. *Wisdom of the Plant Devas* defines how we become our own healers in connection with others who are also their own healers. The premise is one of mutual empowerment and co-creation.

It is also my intention that this book be an inspiration for living more fully and consciously in the present moment. It is here, in the moment, that the making of a story—and the living of it—takes place. The present moment is where the grandest discovery is made and the greatest teaching revealed. May the wisdom of the devas inspire and guide you as together we create a new story and a New Earth.

Acknowledgments

The journey of writing this book has been a stretch between left-brain research and analysis and right-brain creativity and expression. Somewhere in between I dropped into that place where the mind stops and something much greater steps in. For this I am deeply grateful to the devas for appearing in my world and allowing me into theirs. I would also like to thank the staff at Inner Traditions, Bear & Company for the part they are playing in the evolution of consciousness and for empowering our choices through the dissemination of practical and esoteric knowledge. You have affirmed my voice and that of the devas who speak through me, and you have provided the platform from which these voices can be shared.

From the center of my Medicine Wheel Garden, I would like to thank the following for your invaluable encouragement and support: Betsy Sandlin, Susun Weed, Pam Hyde-Nakai, Willie Whitefeather, Matilda Essig, Judith Kaiser, Judith Corvin-Blackburn, Joyce Oliver, Maureen Alvord, Karen Smith, Brad Collins, Lewis Mehl-Madrona, Beverly "Laughing Eagle-Noble Wolf" Martz, Gay Hunter, Colin Wilcox Paxton, Scott Paxton, Nancy Hatcher, and George Poirier. And to all the people who have been in my life at some point in time and nurtured the seeds of my creativity, I carry you with me still.

I would also like to thank my beautiful daughter, Lauren Nicole Loiacono, who "gets" the devas; Sorrel Madrona for the medicine name of Summer Deer; Andy Spraggins for the herbs, deer meat, apples, and hand drumming; Keiya for receiving me as a mother and for teaching me about the sacred feminine through belly dance; Marion Z. Skydancer, whose images inspired my vision of the devas; Adam Bruce Caddick for loving the herbs and my daughter; Jenny Bird for quiet sacred space to write and reflect on a mesa sea of sage and light; Bonnie Marie Poulin for setting me on the journey to find Hanuman; Prem Rawat for knowledge, Barbara Waters for helping me to celebrate the coyotes in my life and the Frank Waters Foundation for nurturing my creative spirit; Laura Cerwinske, sister, friend, and writing coach, who set me on this path from the beginning; Star Wolf for running ahead of the pack, nose to the ground, heart to the wind, and eyes to the heavens; Anyaa McAndrew, sister, friend, and mentor, who has the best taste in chocolate, for embodying sacred marriage with her beloved Gary Stamper; Yellow Horse Man for honoring my medicine and for his medicine of the heart; Grandma Red Leaf for holding the vision of "going to water"; and most important, my heartfelt gratitude to Patricia Kyritsi Howell, registered herbalist, for your mentoring, friendship, and many hours of expert botanical editing that has supported me personally and the publication of this book.

With the exception of the chapter on sagebrush, (which was written on the mesa above the Rio Grande), this book was written in two very sacred places where I have been blessed to live and to grow a garden. It is to the spirit of these places that I humbly bow: Honey Bear Mountain on the Blue Ridge Divide and Isis Cove in the Cherokee Qualla Boundary.

I also wish to acknowledge the new technologies, without which the writing of this book would have been very difficult at best and impossible at worst, as well as the herbalists, writers, and explorers on the edge of evolution who inspired this work, including, but not limited to, the three Barbaras: Barbara Marx Hubbard, Barbara Hand Clow, and Barbara Marciniak.

There is one person without whom this book could not have been conceived, let alone birthed. He is affectionately known as the GreenMan, and he is my foundation, love, and inspiration. It is with all my love that I give gratitude to Charles E. Willhide.

Introduction

*Look deep into nature and then you will understand
everything better.*

ALBERT EINSTEIN

*Nobody sees a flower, really, it is so small. We haven't time—
and to see takes time like to have a friend takes time.*

GEORGIA O'KEEFFE

An exciting field of herbal medicine has appeared on the horizon. Not really
new at all, Earth-Spirit Medicine is being rediscovered at the same time it
is evolving to meet our current physical and spiritual needs. Partially based
on ancient systems of divination and previously available only to the initiated, Earth Spirit Medicine operates on all of the planes between heaven and
earth: physical, spiritual, mental, and emotional. It opens the door to other
dimensions, where we discover not only how powerful the plants are, but also
how powerful *we* are in connection to the divine. At our current evolutionary crossroad we are in need of such a bridge between the physical and the
spiritual, the worlds of botanical medicine and spiritually based medicine, for
in truth these worlds have never been, nor will they ever be, separate.

Herbal medicine takes time. The longest lasting result from ingesting herbs
is obtained from their tonic ability to restore bodily systems: nervous system,
digestive system, circulatory system, and so on. Tonics can be tinctures, teas,

1

extracts, infusions, or decoctions that are taken over periods of time, usually from one to six months. The Heroic and Mechanistic models of healing are popular partially because we want it quick and we want it now. But healing takes time and happens in the context of relationship. It takes time to build relationships. To develop a meaningful and lasting relationship with the healing herbs and their devas is no different. Perhaps that is why the Wise Woman Tradition more accurately describes this model of healing. It takes time to gain wisdom.

If you chose only one herb and really got to know it, you would have a powerful ally. The failure of herbal medicine in many people's experience, or mind, is not a failure at all. It is simply an issue of lack of compliance. To heal with herbal medicine, commitment and consistency are required. In most cases it is not a quick fix. The mindset that says, "If you have this symptom, take this herb," is nothing more than a rephrasing of the Mechanistic model's solution to illness, "If you have this symptom, take this drug." If you make a commitment to yourself and to the herbs, and if you are consistent, you will be richly rewarded on your journey with them. This is also true when working with the spiritual energies of herbs and their devas. The commitment is made in the present moment, one moment at a time, and that commitment becomes a constant flow of energy and intimacy that deepens as you progress. Once you step into this kind of a relationship, healing is a given. While physically ingesting an herb is grounding, once we become spiritually grounded in relationship with the essence of an herb, physically ingesting it becomes secondary and, in some cases, not even necessary.

Within the field of herbal medicine, many labels are used to define a traditional or folk medicine practice: herbalism, herbal medicine, botanical medicine, medical herbalism, herbology, and phytotherapy. Prior to the folk tradition, however, was the shamanic tradition. When this tradition was sent underground, it was the midwives who carried the knowledge of the shamanic tradition forward. They preserved and even expanded that knowledge through the use of their herbs and through journeys into the spirit world and the subconscious mind. It is from this vast, rich resource of the subconscious that higher guidance is obtained.

While traditional herbal medicine does offer a way to discover new healing applications for herbs, research has been primarily focused on identifying botanical compounds and using them in isolation from the whole plant. Even though these medicines are derived from natural sources and are used in a similar manner as with folk medicine, something very vital is missing: synergy. The future of botanical medicine lies in rediscovering methods for using the plant in its whole form, all the elements that go into its creation, including the sacred element of ether.

In part 2, "The Devas: The Architects of Life," we meet and learn who and what the devas are, and how they create in the world of matter. They are in relationship with the elementals, who provide the raw materials for the construction of form. In the chapter titled "The Elementals," new concepts for the dimensions we are time traveling through are presented. This leads us into the "Medicine Wheel Garden," about a multidimensional garden where we become co-creators with nature and magic happens.

The wisdom expressed in part 2 of this book, "The Herbs," is a synthesis of information that weaves our accumulated knowledge of herbs together with awakened consciousness. This would not be possible without the pioneers of science, whose explorations led them to discover, isolate, and label the active ingredients of plants, or those practitioners of the Heroic model of medicine who helped make a wide variety of manufactured herbal medicines available, or the shamans who know how to talk with plants. Nor would it have been possible without all the spiritual teachers who have aspired to lift humanity to a higher octave. The information gathered in the herb chapters, much of it not found compiled anywhere else, serves to ground the spiritual insights as well as to honor all that has come before. The more grounded we become, the more easily we tune into the spiritual realms of the herbs. This attunement will lead us beyond the synthesis of information that is the story we have been telling ourselves about the plants and into the imaginative world of the devas, where a new story of humanity is created.

There can be no doubt that we are remembering how to listen to the voices of the plants. From the accounts in Pam Montgomery's book *Plant Spirit Healing;* Machaelle Small Wright's *Behaving as if the God in All Life Mattered;* Eliot Cowan's *Plant Spirit Medicine;* Paul Hawken's *Magic of Findhorn,* first published in 1975; and Susun Weed's teaching stories in the Wise Woman Tradition, we are reclaiming the ancient wisdom that informed our understanding long before there was a scientific method. When we add the incredible insights given to us by science to the empirical knowledge of older traditions, and then infuse that combination with the empowerment that comes from trusting one's own internal guidance, we create a new model for healing.

Each of the herb chapters in *Wisdom of the Plant Devas* contains three sections that represent past, present, and future, or the fourth dimension of time that we are currently integrating. The first section is called "The Story." It consists of what we know thus far about these healing herbs through our history of interaction with them. In a sense, it is the story of our past, as it contains history and folklore surrounding these herbs. It also includes modern and traditional uses, botanical descriptions, and herbal actions, as well as the common and botanical name, which has its roots in the work of Carl Linnaeus. No matter what opinion one might have about scientific or folk taxonomies, the naming of these plants is a significant part of their story. While it is important to observe a plant as part of a living system without reducing it to merely a name, it is also uniquely human to call something by name. To call something by name keeps it alive in our hearts and in our minds.

Storytelling is a very old form of hypnosis and as such is a powerful tool for transformation. Stories by nature can be contradictory, and it is through the telling, not the resolution, that we come to accept the harmony in the contradiction of our lives. We are being given the opportunity to find the truth for ourselves, even if it contradicts the prewritten scripts. And while it is important that we tell our stories, it is also important not to become overly identified with them. The stories of our past may appear to be written in stone, but they, too, shall eventually return to source as we create yet another story.

The second section is called "The Divination." Here the story of the past informs a higher understanding of how a plant heals and guides us. The focus is on the journey itself from a multidimensional perspective that marries where we've been with where we're going in the ever-present now. It invites us in to the Medicine Wheel Garden and the present moment, where integration takes place. This is where the plant spirit is consulted and herbal medicine takes on a new dimension. "The Divination" is the bridge between "The Story" and "The Deva Speaks," the third and final section. It is also a bridge between what is known and what is unknown, or not yet written, for what is unknown lives both in the future, which is not yet formed, and in our subconscious. We are only just beginning to tap in to the vast jewels of knowledge that live in the storehouse of our subconscious, and we are just learning to trust that knowledge. As we move from the darkness of the unknown, we take in the elementals from the rich soil of our existence. Just as a seed pushes up through the earth, we move into the light of what is known, and a greater story emerges.

The Deva Speaks section contains my transcription of the channeled voice of each herb deva, charged with a power beyond the informational value of the words. Direct from the world of spirit, these are timely messages for personal growth and planetary transformation. These messages inspire us to find our own personal truths and give us the tools for exploring our psyches. This is the Medicine for a New Earth. At this time, when we stand in the galactic center of our universe and experience the shift of the ages, we will move out of the control frequency (for example, controlling what herbs may or may not be made available to us) and into the world of illumination, where we have everything we need at any given moment. This is what the herbs *and* their devas have to teach us.

Each chapter in part 2, "The Herbs," is complete unto itself. They can be read in any order and used as a divination tool merely by opening to any chapter. Herbs have not only internal physiological effects, but spiritual and psychological dimensions as well. Addressing them in this way encourages communication with the subconscious, as the devas teach us how to listen, not only to the herbs, but also to ourselves. In the words of Eliot Cowan, "The magic is not in the matter. It's in the spirit." There is also a section, in the very back of the book, titled "Herbal Actions," which is another useful tool to educate you about the specific effects that herbs have on the body.

The discussions throughout this book on political concerns and varying topics of alternative and energetic medicine are not conclusive and are meant only to provide an introduction to these topics along with insights and resources. And while many philosophical and metaphysical concepts are presented throughout this book, it is not necessary to hold any particular cultural or spiritual belief to benefit from reading it. While most of these concepts are not presented in great depth, as that would require filling volumes, they serve as keys to open our hearts and minds to a greater truth about who we really are. The exploration of these concepts in further depth is the journey of discovery you will hopefully be inspired to make as your soul is awakened and your consciousness expanded.

While the pioneering holistic health fields of vibrational medicine are breaking ground in addressing issues of emotional well-being, soul development, and mind-body health through disciplines like homeopathy, flower essences, and plant spirit medicine, we are at the point where the next step that is required of us will be a quantum leap. We have broken the components of our world down into smaller and smaller fragments in order to understand how it works and to create new things, but this reductionism has only made us more fragmented. This is not a bad thing, but actually a blessing that is leading us to the realization that mystics, saints, and yogis have always known: all matter exists in a unified field of consciousness from which we are not separate. This holographic field exists as much inside of us as we exist in it. We are creator beings learning about our next level of creative abilities within this universe of possibilities. But a shift is necessary and inevitable in order for us to fully step into this next level. It is a shift into our light bodies, bodies that resonate at a higher frequency than our temporal bodies. The miracle is that we can experience that light and the knowledge of the source of all things while we are still in a physical body. It is through this direct experience that we find the doors of perception opening to the libraries of time: past, present, and future. It is a resonance phenomenon. The more we align with these higher truths, the more we resonate with them, and the more we resonate with them, the more our soul awakens, and the more our soul awakens, the more we step into being our Higher Selves.

Imagine a New Earth where survival is no longer a concern. Where our emotions are fluid, we are sovereign unto ourselves, and we know ourselves as creator. Where we are aligned with our intuition and inner knowing while following our inner guidance. Imagine traveling at the speed of thought. When consciousness becomes fully infused in matter, we will transcend time and space and come home to love. The New Earth awaits us. We are limited in physical form only by the laws that govern this dimension, but our consciousness is limited only by our perception and knows no bounds. The devas understand this evolution of consciousness that is the liberator of material form. They are holding open the door.

The Devas

The Architects of Life

In the Garden of the Devas

The human evolution should give strength to the deva, and the deva, joy to the human.

ALICE A. BAILEY, *LETTERS ON OCCULT MEDITATION*

Devas exist throughout all of nature as the architects of life. As we playfully explore in the Garden of the Devas, you will be amazed at what they have so patiently been waiting for us to discover. This garden exists wherever and whenever you find yourself opening to nature and seeing the world through new eyes with an awareness of the devas who created it. They are the unseen, other side of nature, responsible for keeping everything alive. Without them we could not survive. Although they may go unseen to the untrained eye, devas joyfully appear in their luminous form to the clairvoyant and may even be heard by the clairaudient.

The word *deva* is a Sanskrit word meaning "body of light" or "shining one." In Buddhism, devas are compassionate beings who live in the higher realms but are still subject to the laws of rebirth. Various texts regarding devas seem to closely associate them with faeries and angels, but they are not mythical wee folk, those who act as intermediaries with the spirit world, or messengers of God. They work on an etheric level to orchestrate the energies that create the specific forms of nature. Devas hold all of the cellular blueprints and genetic codes for plants in their memories. A plant's deva can bring even a plant species that has become "extinct" back into this dimension when a great need for its specific medicine is determined. Every herb, fruit, flower, and vegetable has its own deva, its own identity, and its own character. Devas have been embraced, it seems, by every culture and given many names. The Jews called this energy *Ruach Elohim;* the Egyptians, *Gengen Wer;* the Persians, *Devs;* and the Dinka tribe in Africa, *Abuk.* You have only to ask them, by whatever name, to learn what they have to teach.

Everything in nature is endowed with intelligence and spirit. When we are in communication with the devas, we enter into a deeper relationship with the spirit of the plants. When we are in touch with a plant's spirit, we are more receptive to information about its medicine. In this time of rampant destruction of planetary resources, the devas hold the keys to rapid restoration. Because healing takes place within the context of relationship, they desire our human interaction to accomplish this. We are the ones who must carry out the wisdom they are all too eager to share with us. By becoming more aware of the role that the devas play in our everyday lives, we not only heal on a physical level but also may discover that the strongest medicine lies in their ability to help us to heal our hearts, our minds, and our spirits. Every time we receive the healing essence of a plant, we also receive communion.

Everything we know about medicine we learned in one way or another from plants. No surgery, diagnosis, or remedy would be accomplished without the evolution of knowledge acquired through our relationship with plants. Surgery requires drugs, which are derived from plants. Diagnosis takes observation, which was practiced by our ancestors in their observations of the natural world. Appropriate remedies were prescribed based on these observations and adjusted according to what worked or didn't work. All of this has been accomplished through our relationship with plants, a relationship that requires deep trust, patience, and time. Remedies based on observation, diagnosis, and prescription are part of a medical model that originated in folk medicine. Folk medicine, or natural medicine, relies heavily on a working knowledge of plants. We are utterly dependent on plants for all of our basic needs—from shelter, fuel, and clothing to medicine and food.

In the Garden of the Devas you will find communities living together in much the same manner as we do. Devic communities may include nature spirits, faeries, and elementals. While the devas pass the "blueprints" to the nature spirits, who in turn construct the form from the raw materials provided by the elementals, the faeries direct and guide the work of the nature spirits. The faeries are overseen by the elementals, who govern earth, water, fire, and air. This orchestrated dance is always changing and never static. It could look like many things as we shift our consciousness into the next dimension and the magical world of the devas. We are all perfectly playing our evolutionary roles. There is no higher or lower, merely a spectrum of degrees of separation. Devic communities have established not a hierarchy, but a society in which they are learning how to work and grow together, all with their own special talent and gift. They have been at this much longer than we, the people, have. Everything and all the entities of Mother Earth are related, and we are all learning how to better work together to create a beautiful garden.

One of the ways we could create a garden might look like this: A landscape architect (deva) develops a plan or layout for the garden. The helpers or those employed by the architect (faeries) direct and guide the gardeners (nature spirits) in the execution of the plan. The nature spirits prepare the soil; bury the seeds; water and maintain the plants as they grow; and weed, edge, trim, and prune to create a beautiful and aesthetic garden.

With the help and guidance of the faeries, the nature spirits tend to the garden. Prayers are then made to the elementals, whom they humbly ask to bring favorable conditions for growth. These prayers are answered in the form of the earth element becoming fertile soil facilitated by microorganisms and being made ready to receive the seeds. Seeds, the rewards of flowering and bearing fruit, are carried by the wind, the element of air. The element of water, like our own emotions, waters the bodies, and roots, of plant and flesh. The fire element of our sun lives within each one of us and is the very essence of life. For the plants, chlorophyll made in partnership with the sun is akin to our own blood. It is how the energy of light is processed into chemical energy, which can then be stored in the body. The same mechanism is true for us and is what allows our eyes to process light into nerve signals. A theme that seems to repeat when the devas speak is that of a Central Sun that illuminates the vision of our soul. Nature spirits call to the elementals much as our spirits are calling now: for water, earth, fire, and air. We long for connection to that from which we came.

Earth Keepers, people who own or care for land with the intention of preserving it for the next seven generations, appreciate the beauty, health, and ease that comes from leaving a piece of land to nature's hand. Beauty is truly in the eye of the beholder. May we behold the beauty of both the wild and cultivated places, for both are necessary for our continuation.

Madame Helena P. Blavatsky, cofounder of the Theosophical Society in 1875, introduced her own ideas about devas to the West. She believed they came to Earth before the elementals and remained dormant until we reached a certain stage of our human evolution. Then, the devas joined with the elementals to help further our spiritual development. If there was ever a time when we needed to call on the devas, it is now. We have penetrated the wildest places and climbed the highest peaks, but we have yet to seek the life within the form or to scale the heights of our own consciousness.

Even though devas live a very long time, they evolve just as we do. When their work is complete, they move on, and when it is not, they are reborn in yet another form, albeit a light body, to continue their work and evolution. While it may look like we are facing unprecedented mass extinctions, the world of nature balances itself in a dynamic disequilibrium. To say that something is in a "state of balance" does not mean that it is static. There is always movement and a counterbalancing between the opposites. Not only is everything connected and related within this dimension, everything is connected throughout all worlds and all dimensions. We are seeing and learning from the results of our choices, and nature is balancing the effects of those choices with her perfect wisdom. What is important to remember is that we have a choice, and we are always making the best choices possible given the resources we have available. The devas hold the key to unlocking our ability to increase and mobilize resources. At this time many of the devas are choosing to evolve to another dimension.

Many humans are also now choosing to evolve, with this being their last incarnation on this plane of existence. This evolution of consciousness is leading us toward the creation of a New Earth. This has been expressed in the Hopi prophesies as the end of the Fourth World of separation and the beginning of the Fifth World of illumination. What exists within each and every one of us, at the very core of the atoms of which we are made, is pure energy, pure light.

The devas, who are already in their light bodies, are guiding and supporting us as we enter the New Earth, warmed by a Central Sun. What this Central Sun is, we do not yet know, as it lives beyond four-dimensional reality. What we do know is that our solar sun warms our physical bodies from without, and the Central Sun is a light that warms our souls from within. The spiritual Masters have taught us that we can see this light when our third eye is open. Meditation techniques and yoga practices teach us how to access this light, which is activated through the pineal gland. The devas facilitate a similar activation when we take the time to call on their wisdom.

Now, at this momentous time in our human history, aided by the devas, who *are* the Ascended Masters, we are being given the opportunity to birth a New Earth, one which will herald the end of the fossil age and the beginning of the solar age. Ecclesiastes 1:9 describes the Old Earth from which we are ascending: "The thing that hath been, it is that which shall be; and that which is done is that which shall be done: and there is no new thing under the sun." This statement accurately describes consciousness, as it presently exists in what will become known as the Old Earth. For what has been is what shall be until we shift our consciousness beyond what is presently perceived.

By coming into community with the devas and the world of nature that exists around and inside of us, and by calling on the wisdom of the medicine plants, we gain tremendous insights that will ultimately ease the transition into the next dimension.

The devas are perfectly poised to give us these insights. They are giving us the keys to unlock our imagination and our heart. Even the caterpillar that completely dissolves in order to become something wholly new holds in its imagination the seed of another form. The more we learn how to communicate with the unseen worlds, the more we will strengthen our inner knowing and come to trust our own inner guidance system. If ever there was a time to seek this guidance, it is *now*. In discovering who we really are and for what greater purpose we have been born, all beings in all dimensions are lifted up.

May you be perfectly guided by the devas through all the seasons of your life.

The Elementals

Yet there is a profound truth, namely this: When man loses the heavens, he loses himself. By far the most important elements of man's being belong to the universe beyond the Earth and if he loses sight of this universe he loses sight of his own true being. He wanders over the Earth without knowing what kind of being he really is.

RUDOLF STEINER, "COSMIC FORCES IN MAN"
LECTURE, OSLO, NOVEMBER 24, 1921

The ninety-two natural chemical elements that we know of thus far are the raw materials used to make everything we find here on Earth. These chemical elements are also contained within the classical elements of earth, air, fire, and water, also known as the elemental clans. But there is a fifth element that is not made up of these chemical elements, but is responsible for activating them, and it is called ether. This fifth sacred thing is the realm of spirit. It is the realm where the devas live and conceive the world. It is a world that is not only totally dependent on the elementals, but would not survive or even be possible without them.

The elements are made up of different kinds of atoms, and at the core of every atom is light. The chemical elements that science has so far classified, including the ones that make up our bodies, were created in the supernova explosions of dying stars. There is ancient knowledge encoded in these bits of stardust. Even the five elements of water, wood, fire, earth, and metal used in Chinese medicine describe something much older than what is presently understood. These elements contain *qi*, or the life force energy that animates all things. The great Hermetic Principle "as above, so below; as within, so without" rings with the universal truth that we are literally made of and governed by stars. Each plant whose body is built from the raw materials of the elements and whose form was conceived by the devas is connected to the stars, no different than we are.

This view of the human as being of the whole cosmos is rooted in many ancient traditions and philosophies. It was expounded in the work of Rudolf Steiner,* one of history's most original thinkers, and his ongoing legacy continues to provide us with a bridge between science and spirit, and between heaven and earth. Plants and humans as they relate to each other and the cosmos didn't evolve separately, but concurrently. One of the ways to view this is through the lens of interconnectedness. The elementals have placed themselves within us and within the plants that sustain us. Our world is literally constructed from the elementals, according to the blueprint of the devas. What exists within us exists in nature, and what exists in nature is also within us. An example of this would be the foxglove plant, which produces digitalis. We also produce digitalis, and because of this we are inextricably linked to this plant. In our nervous system we have opiates called endorphins that exist in nature in the form of the poppy plant. Inside of us we have hormones that are also produced in plants. One could even say that we produce these plants within us, yet we continue to search outside for what already lies within.

There are thousands of substances that exist outside of us that our bodies also produce. This is the foundation for the intimate relationship between plant and human in which healing takes place. The devas present us with this reoccurring theme: *healing takes place in the context of relationships*. It is not necessary to strive for harmonious relationships, for we are already in

---

*Rudolf Steiner is one the most significant occultists to come forward in the past century. He founded the spiritual movement anthroposophy, based on a philosophy that brings the spiritual traditions of central Europe into a modern context where direct experience of a spiritual world is accessible through meditation and inner development. He also developed Waldorf education, biodynamic agriculture, and anthroposophical medicine, based on this philosophy. Steiner was influenced by the work of Goethe and Nietzsche, and wrote books about their work. Despite Steiner's extensive works, he is still largely unknown in the world today.

harmony with the world around us. It is in the striving that we separate our-selves from the glorious knowledge of our interconnectedness. Healing is not a rational process.

By ingesting plants, either spiritually or physically, we can recalibrate the body so that it remembers how to optimally function. This is what the devas call the "original instructions of Creator." The elements in plants communi-cate with the elements in our bodies through a resonant field. We are only just beginning to understand field phenomena and how we affect the world around us through thought, sympathetic resonance, and morphogenetic fields. The imaginal cells in insect larvae are examples of morphogenetic fields. The electromagnetic fields explored by Marcel Vogel* in his experiments with crystals showed us the power of a crystal to store, amplify, convert, and cohere subtle energies. He discovered what the mystics have always known: love is the cohering force. The elementals are oscillators similar to crystals. Crystals can be programmed to vibrate at a certain frequency and then bring us into a corresponding frequency.

The elementals can also be programmed and are being programmed by humans and by the devas. We in turn program the world around us through our vibrational frequency. The human body is also like a crystal oscillator that vibrates in time between two different states. In this example we might say that we are vibrating between states of consciousness. Currently we are electromagnetic water beings and as such can be programmed by sound and light, which is how the devas are programming us along with the elementals that live within us.

We vibrate at a specific frequency, just like a crystal, creating a resonance and emitting an electrical signal. These frequencies are commonly used to keep track of time or to transmit and receive radio signals. The signals that we transmit and receive are part of a grid system that creates a circuit around our crystalline structure. This crystalline structure is a part of our Earth and our physical bodies. As we struggle to grasp the concept of higher dimensions of

---

*Marcel Vogel's areas of expertise were phosphor technology as it relates to luminescence in crystalline structures, liquid crystal systems, and magnetics. In the 1970s Vogel did pioneer-ing work in man-plant communication experiments. This led him to the study of quartz crystals.

space and time, the ideas presented in this book may be helpful in the integration of a higher understanding of who and what we are, and in the creating of a foundation from which to vision our lives.

I think everyone would agree that we are living in a three-dimensional physical reality governed by duality. We could also say that this is a three-dimensional universe, or a physical plane of existence in the third dimension. The popular string theory of matter holds that there are three dimensions we perceive as space and one dimension of time, the fourth. We share the common dimensions of space, which is governed by the laws of nature.

The discussion of multidimensional reality in this book is based on existing theories, and at the same time it is a new theory of the dimensions of space and time as informed by the wisdom of the plant devas. One of these theories is that of Einstein's relativity and the identification of time as the fourth dimension. Einstein's work is still unfolding, and it would be interesting to note that I was born the year he died. One question I have repeatedly asked myself in this lifetime, from the depths of my soul, is, "What is time?" Einstein was searching for a unification theory based on general relativity and a continuous view of the universe. But a problem arises when we try to perceive or understand something, in this case another dimension, that is beyond the one we are currently experiencing because we are limited by our tools of perception as defined by that dimension. Only by fully entering the present moment may we transcend this limitation and expand our consciousness.

Time, as it has been revealed by the devas, exists both in and as the fourth dimension, but at present we only experience the linear portion as it projects into three-dimensional space, not unlike the way we project three-dimensional objects onto two-dimensional space. Time as we perceive it in the fourth dimension is linear, but in truth it is nonlinear. We do not yet live fully in the fourth dimension, and once this dimension is fully integrated we will see that all time—past, present, and future—exists simultaneously on the spiral ladder of evolution.

While humans evolved from the elementals, who are vibrating between the second and third dimensions, those of us who are choosing to evolve consciousness are now oscillating between the third and fourth dimensions because we are tuning ourselves to the higher frequencies as we prepare to

shift into the fifth dimension and evolve into our light bodies. This is happening due to the increase of light on the planet from both our solar sun
and from our expanding consciousness. The devas are currently oscillating
between four- and five-dimensional consciousness in preparation for their
leap into the worlds that will be made available to them. The fifth dimension
therefore becomes space-time, no separation, only illumination. A metaphor
for what this oscillation might look like from our limited perspective of four-
dimensional reality is spiritual bungee cord jumping. As we raise our vibrational frequency, we are learning to program the elementals in the same way
that the devas do—through the cohering force of love.

The element of phosphorus is the light bearer in the mineral world, and
deprived of light we get sick. Elemental phosphorus is a component in DNA
and an essential element for all living cells. As the light shifts and increases,
the parts of our DNA that have lain dormant also shift and become activated.
The word *phosphorus* is derived from Greek mythology and means "light-
bearer." The name Lucifer has the same meaning, and it is derived from the
Latin *lux,* meaning "light," and *fer,* meaning "bearing." Lucifer refers to the
Morning Star, or Venus, who is the goddess of love and beauty. *Lucifer* and
phosphorus literally mean "bringer of light." This kind of esoteric and alchemical knowledge was lost when the meaning behind the words was twisted to
serve the religious and political power agendas that sought to retain control
over the masses. The light of love illuminates all things, transforms all things,
and brings us closer to a New Earth.

We know that light deprivation results in weakness and poor cellular
growth. Reunited with light through the sun, crystals, or plants, our cellular
structure is restored. When the body gets taken over by microbes, it is no
different than when a weak plant gets taken over by fungus in order to be
recycled back into nature. This is an example of the oscillation that is taking
place between the second and third dimensions. A weak plant, like a weak
human, has diminished light and life-force energy and is no longer vibrant.
This change in structural form results in a transformation to a more appropriate form based on elemental composition. As long as we are oscillating
between the third and fourth dimensions, and not stuck in time or space,
we are not affected by the loss of life-force energy, even as the body is being

returned to the earth, for our spirit retains its vibrancy as it travels back into the ether, and life-force energy is transferred through the crystalline structures of the elementals into another vehicle of physical expression.

If we paid closer attention to the qualities of vibrancy and life-force energy, how different would the choices be that we make with regard to what surrounds us or goes into our bodies? How much closer would we be to vibrating at the frequency of light? When illness becomes the enemy instead of the effort to restore balance to the body, we have lost sight of how to guide the body through illness to its healthful conclusion. This is true on all levels when we make anything an enemy to be fought against. We have lost our guides and been taught to live in fear of the wild and unpredictable power of nature, a power that has the ability to heal. The wisdom to support the body to express through illness with medicine rather than to suppress through knowledge of pharmaceuticals is the difference between healing and heroics. Medicine in this context becomes whatever supports healing: physical, spiritual, or otherwise.

When a child becomes ill and is lovingly guided through the chaos of a fever and infection, then healing occurs. The fever is not the offender, nor is the infection. They serve only to expel the offender. The offender is not an invader to be defended against. If the child's immune system is repressed, then an acute symptom turns into a chronic pattern. The goal is to see an illness to its natural conclusion, which is a restoration of health, just as the earth is restored after the hard, cold expression of winter and the erratic expression of spring. The earth doesn't defend herself against winter; she merely makes adjustments and is supported by the elementals to do so. When the body is not supported to heal itself and see illness through to its natural conclusion, disease results, and sometimes this can occur through generations of genetically encoded imbalance. But where are our guides to healing? Who will sit patiently by our bedsides and administer the medicine? And what will be our medicine?

The indigenous peoples of Earth have always understood how this principle of healing works and what it means to let nature take its course. We can no longer think our way through life or an illness. There's more to it than that. Thinking allows us to perceive only ideas, while the intelligence of nature allows us to perceive the universe.

Each one of us has an individual and unique experience with life and the elementals from which we are made. For example, one person may have experienced living through the elemental force of a hurricane, while another may have survived a very cold night lost in the wilderness. These experiences heighten our awareness and bring us a little closer to that part of ourselves that is not separate from nature. Just as each of us experiences the elementals in a different way, each of us experiences the devas through our individual filters and life experiences. What is important is that we allow the devas to live in our imagination and that we nurture our relationship with them. As our awareness of the devas increases and we learn to listen and communicate with them, they will teach us about our relationship to the elementals and to ourselves. The elementals teach us about where we came from and where we are going. Each plant is a unique individual, just as each human being is a unique individual, and no two interactions will be the same.

THE DEVA SPEAKS

To the elementals of my heart, I would say that my love for you is the most profound. You come from the stars that are born of the void at the creative center of all universes and have given rise to my visions and dreams. I am with you in sacred union and honor you as my beloveds.

To the humans of my heart, I would also say that my love for you is the most profound. While I am made of light and live in the ether, I am a dimensional being as you are, and we serve in each other's evolution. You also are made of light but still live mostly in the darkness of the third dimension and have become comfortable with your dependency on the elementals. It is time for you to learn what I know: the elementals are at your service. They took flight through you as they evolved into three-dimensional existence, and now you, my beloveds, are taking flight and evolving into the dimensions from which I speak. You are in service to the evolution of consciousness.

One of the hardest things for you to witness at this time is what you perceive to be the destruction of your Earth. But I will say to you that out of this destruction the New Earth is being created. It is in the dissolution of form that new forms are created. You have chosen this path of learning by your own free will, and as your consciousness grasps the gift of grace that lies beyond the lessons, you near the completion of your journey. When you become aware that nothing is created in your universe except from the raw materials already at hand and provided to you, as they are to me, by the elementals, you will bring forth creations that are more soundly based on the laws of matter and form. It is from the elementals that you will learn to create on higher levels. It is impossible for you to destroy them, and you are only just now learning to see them as they really are—and yourselves for who you really are. The destruction of the creations of your world is the result of how you have used the elementals. This was necessary for you to develop an understanding of this elemental world and the part of you that it reflects. You are infinite beings of light, and your darkness exists only to nurture the seed from which a new form will emerge. All things are conceived in the darkness of the void and emerge from it, even the elementals, from which all things are made. Know that the light of consciousness is dawning and your way is illuminated, as together in sacred union we conceive, and birth, the New Earth.

The Medicine Wheel Garden

As women have become afraid of the experience of birthing their own kind into being, the Goddess has been tricked into fearing her greatest ability: to bring forth and nurture life.

BARBARA MARCINIAK, *FAMILY OF LIGHT*

In Tibetan medicine the ideal garden is not seen as existing on Earth, but within the four directions between four medicine mountains. It is a heavenly garden that nestles in valleys thicketed with wildflowers and medicinal plants among pools of crystal-clear water. All creatures living in this wild and beautiful garden anchor the celestial influences within it, and none are ever harmed. In the land of the Navajo, we also see four medicine mountains in the four sacred directions, where the three sacred rivers flow into one and hold the healing songs of a people who grow corn, beans, and squash. Whether a heavenly world above or an earthly world below, the magical garden, until now, has somehow seemed to live only at the edge of our consciousness.

What is changing as a result of our evolving consciousness is that the Medicine Wheel Garden is coming into focus as the illusion of separation dissolves. It is a garden that lives in the magical realms between heaven and earth, and between human and deva. The Medicine Wheel Garden as it exists on Earth is a three-dimensional representation of the "as above, so below" mysteries. It is in the shape of a circle that contains a six-pointed star, and it is a mirror of the heavens. As it sits on the earth in three-dimensional reality, it represents the six directions: east, south, west, north, above, and below. Within this garden grows all the food and medicine that sustains us in our current form while simultaneously feeding our evolution into our light bodies.

The Medicine Wheel is an ever-turning circle that contains within it the whole of creation. It is a universal symbol, a sacred hoop that teaches us about the interconnectedness of life. Ancient stone circles have been found on every continent, marking territorial and celestial influences. These circles or wheels create a vortex where we receive guidance from the devas on our earth walk. The Medicine Wheel Garden is the fertile place where we can go, a sacred space in our backyards, in our homes, or in our imaginations to connect with something greater than ourselves, a place to meditate, pray, and envision a New Earth, for it is through our imagination that we create whole new worlds. A Medicine Wheel becomes a Medicine Wheel Garden when we imbue it with life. This can be done simply by being present in a space and breathing, for it is our breath that animates the spirit.

There are two kinds of medicine: elemental medicine and ether medicine. Elemental medicine mends our ills through the benefits of earth, air, fire, and water. Earth medicine heals our bodies, air our minds, fire our passions, and water our emotions. Plants contain all of these elements, and we also find them in four of the six directions of the Medicine Wheel Garden. Ether medicine heals with essence. It lives at the center of the Medicine Wheel Garden. The fifth sacred element, ether, is the most basic element of our existence. It is the essence of love. Ether medicine exists in the place where we began and the place we shall return. It encompasses the other two directions of above and below to create the seventh direction of "within" that is sometimes referred to in certain tribal Medicine Wheel teachings. Both medicines can heal us, but it is in the marrying of the elemental and devic worlds that new worlds are born. The elementals' presence in the third dimension is because they have been lifted up from the second dimension through human evolution. Everything that exists in the third dimension is an expression of the elementals. Humanity is oscillating between the third and fourth dimensions and is being strongly impulsed by the devas.

The Medicine Wheel Garden is an overlay of many systems of healing. It is a grid as well as a map. It exists in this dimension and many others simultaneously, for it holds all of creation within it and is a mirror of the cosmos. This is one of the reasons we are seeing so many overlapping concepts in various systems of healing and branches of spirituality, religion, and thought. There are even new names for these systems like "complementary medicine" and "New Thought spirituality." Humanity is expanding to include a larger vision of our purpose. Using elemental and ether medicine together, we not only complete the sacred hoop, we also transcend it. The world of duality is represented in these two medicines. Marrying them dissolves the illusion of separateness, but a collective vision is necessary for a new form to emerge. Much like when the caterpillar dissolves in the chrysalis, the imaginal cells hold the vision of the butterfly yet to emerge. We must now hold that vision for a New Earth.

Each direction in the Medicine Wheel Garden brings us a teaching about some aspect of our lives. These teachings are shared with us by the herbs and their devas. As we move further up the spiral ladder of evolution, however, and begin to transcend space and time, these directions become less defined. At the same time that the Medicine Wheel Garden is a container for the whole of life as we know it, it also contains what is beyond our knowing. It is a place where we come into alignment with our Highest Self at the turning of the ages. The Medicine Wheel Garden gives us a reference point from which to begin our journey into multidimensional realities. Everything is mirrored in the Medicine Wheel Garden, and within everything is a Medicine Wheel. We see this in the sacred geometry of the repeating patterns of life and nature. Just as a flower is contained within the Medicine Wheel, so is the Medicine Wheel contained within the flower. We live in a holographic universe.

Within us are great wheels of light that we call the chakra system. All of life, from the great spiral galaxies to the billions of atoms spinning within a grain of sand, is composed of these spinning wheels of light. We ourselves are spinning on the earth around the sun. The Medicine Wheel Garden is a representation of this wheel of life, where we receive and assimilate divine nourishment, and transmit this life-force energy back out into the world. The Medicine Wheel Garden is a wheel within a wheel. The wheel is a fundamental building block of nature and the circle of life that flows through all creation.

The Medicine Wheel Garden is best perceived through the wisdom of the heart. In this garden everything is medicine, and it shows up at the hour of our need. The masculine forces needed at this time to balance the feminine have historically ruled from the head and the feminine forces from the heart. For this reason, women are reclaiming their role as healers among the people, supported by a new masculine energy that understands the role of the feminine and does no harm. Everyone has a medicine gift to carry in this garden. We are here to be in service to the evolution of consciousness and the unfolding of a New Earth.

What waits to be discovered in the Medicine Wheel Garden of the devas is the divinatory nature of plants. When we slow down and perceive with an open heart, we see that each plant within the wheel becomes a tool for divination. The Medicine Wheel Garden is based on one of the reoccurring themes in this book, "as above, so below; as within, so without." Ancient systems of divination are also based on this same premise. The idea that our unconscious is mirrored in our external reality, and the events in our external reality are but mirrors of our internal condition, attracts to us exactly what we need in any given moment. This is also known as the Law of Attraction or the Principle of Correspondence. There are dimensions beyond our knowing, but through this law or principle we can begin to understand what might otherwise be unknowable. Divination is a tool not only for navigating between the known and unknown, but also for mirroring our unconscious back to us. This greatly increases our resources for personal growth and development. Historically, divination has been carried out through interpreting the pulling and laying of cards in spreads, the throwing of stones and bones, and the interpretation of signs.

The popularity of divination during the past few decades has given us an opportunity to practice being divinely guided. It has encouraged communication with the subconscious and taught us how to listen at a deep level. By practicing divination we have become more aware of the signs, or hidden meanings, in a seemingly random set of circumstances. In discovering how to interpret these circumstances, we learn to trust our intuition, our inner guidance, and ultimately our inner authority. As we learn to trust ourselves, we become less dependent on the beliefs of others and more empowered and response-able for our actions. Empowered people make empowered choices, and this serves the highest good of us all.

Soon it will no longer be necessary to receive guidance from clearly defined systems of divination, as everything is being mirrored in our reality moment by moment. The systems were in place merely to teach us how these principles work. Now that we know how they work, it is time to internalize them and apply them at the quantum level. This doesn't mean we don't reach for the oracle cards when confusion sets in; it just means that we have the ability to communicate directly and receive guidance directly from the oracle in all things. As we learn to listen to the still, small voice within, we might find that we are being spoken to in much the same manner that a counselor would speak to us in a therapeutic setting, a counselor who challenges us to find our own inner answers.

As we discover these answers through our interactions with each other and the natural world, we will see that the animals have had much to teach us about our animal bodies and natures. The plants, however, are teaching us about our light bodies, and their complexity exceeds what we previously thought. They are more sensitive to their environment and give rise to faster mutations. Both plants and animals are reaching and surpassing the greatest levels of extinction known, rivaling even that of the dinosaurs. What do plants have to teach us? Everything. Each has a personality and a purpose according to the environment in which it was designed. One of the lessons of the Medicine Wheel Garden that we can take back with us into our everyday lives is that all of life is sacred. The oracle of the medicine plants also teaches us reverence and how to intuit the deeper meaning of our lives.

We all stand at some point in the Medicine Wheel Garden. We all walk the Medicine Wheel of life. We may journey many times around the wheel in this one life, gathering medicine from the six elemental directions: east, south, west, north, above, and below. In this circle there is no end, only cycles of change: conception, incubation, gestation, birth, growth, rise, zenith, decline, death, and decay, then starting all over again. The placement of each stone, each plant, and each step in the Medicine Wheel Garden brings new insight. When we leave our physical incarnation and walk the blue road of spirit from the north of the Medicine Wheel to the east, where life begins again, we walk the Milky Road of our ancestors as we cross the Milky Way. Look deep into the eyes of these ancestors, these stars from which we all have taken our birth. Some lights go out, and some explode into being. We will know all of this and more at the center of the Medicine Wheel Garden.

The roots of our ancestors hold us in the physical plane of existence, much the same way that the roots of the medicine plants hold terra firma in the Medicine Wheel Garden. Plants seek to evolve, just as we do, and the devas are our future ancestors. On our mutual evolutionary journey, we must heal our ancestral lineages so that we may pass beyond the veils of separation. This is one of the reasons it was important to name the families of the herbs that appear in this book. The plants can assist us with this healing when we feel their firm, stout roots tenaciously gripping the earth beneath our feet. If you want to get at the root of a health problem, or any problem for that matter, step into the Medicine Wheel Garden and seek the medicine of roots. The roots hold great medicine for us at this time, and the ancestors want us to heal.

The time has come, and the shift of the ages is upon us. The seeds have been planted in the Medicine Wheel Garden and in our lives, protected by the divine masculine, which sometimes appears in the form of the Green Man, and nurtured by the sacred feminine. We have loved these seeds the best we could, carried and protected them the best we could. And now, through the divination of the medicine plants and the deepening of intimacy between us and the devas, who have been trying very hard to get our attention, our consciousness is expanding beyond our previously perceived limitations. Once we have stepped into the Medicine Wheel Garden, we have entered safe space. All that has been created will be healed here. It is a requirement of healing to feel held and to be safe. When a seed pushes up through the earth, drawn by the warmth and promise of the sun, it is a thrust toward life. We should remember what it is to thrust new life into the world. To bring forth and nurture life is one of our greatest creative abilities.

In her book *Family of Light,* Barbara Marciniak explains that when we unnecessarily cut our babies from our bodies (as in giving birth by caesarean section), we deny them their inherent right to thrust forward into life and hold a frequency of fear for who they might be, rather than welcoming them no matter who they are. We are at a point where we are birthing something wholly new, thrusting toward the light of a Central Sun. We must trust ourselves in the process, surrender, and allow what is coming to emerge. Both masculine and feminine forces are necessary, and we will find great strength in yielding. By entering the Medicine Wheel Garden, connecting with the elements through our roots, and taking communion with the devas, we will learn to trust in our deepest self and have reverence for all of life.

Be who you are. Be where you are. Then have a look around and decide where you want to go. As long as the songs are sung and the stories are told, the land will continue to flourish, and in its flourishing, it will give rise to a New Earth. We all stand in the Medicine Wheel Garden together. Enter . . .

The Song of the 6 Winds

Feels like 6 Winds are ever blowin' me,
through my days, and through my life.
Can I find 6 friends ever showin' me
The way to see the light?

She was a blue wind, blown from yesterday,
and her memory haunts me down.
But you're a new wind, blowin' warm my way
We'll let tomorrow twirl us around.

Look around you now, see the hurricanes
well don't let them blow you away.
Look inside you now, you're a tornado,
and I believe you'll find your way.

Lookin' like 6 Winds are ever blowin',
through your days, and through your lives.
Lookin' like 6 friends ever showin' you
the way to see the light.

High above us all, see our star shine,
may it be our guiding light.
Deep below us all, feel our Earth so fine
we will stand our ground tonight.

Seems like 6 Winds are ever blowin'
through our days and through our lives
I see 6 friends ever showin' us
the way to see the light . . .
And if it's 6 Winds, ever blowin' us,
I believe we'll be all right.
May be 6 Winds ever blowin' us,
but only one heartbeat tonight.

JOHN ROMAN

The Herbs

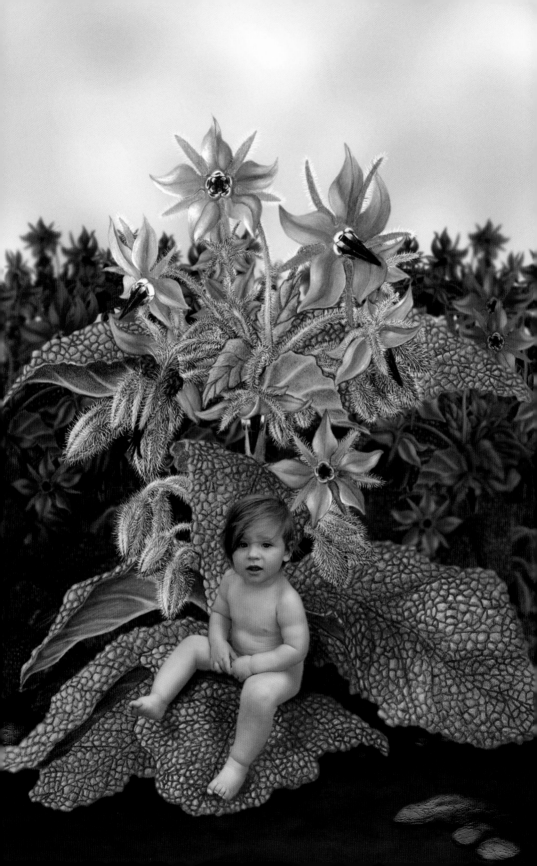

Borage

Borago officinalis

Courage

THE STORY

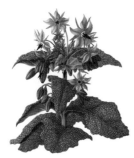

Ancient and mythical, *Borago officinalis* has a five-pointed blue flower and is also known as starflower. It is highly attractive to bees and long prized for its culinary and medicinal qualities. This herb most likely originated in an area known as the Levant, from a Middle French word meaning "the Orient," located in what is now Syria, at the crossroads of western Asia, the eastern Mediterranean, and northeast Africa, an area that has been closely linked with spices throughout its history and whose spice trade included medicinal herbs like borage. Hieroglyphic inscriptions in the Great Temple of Amun at Karnak describe the medical botanical garden of Thutmosis III, which contained plants and flowers from Syria and Arabia. The illustrious Moors, who transformed the dry Spanish plains into rich agricultural areas with their irrigation systems, brought borage to medieval Spain from Syria. From there, borage spread all over Europe and eventually naturalized throughout the world.

The name *borage* has come down to us through the annals of time. In Medieval Latin, it was known as *borrago;* in botanical Latin, *borago;* in Old

31

French, *bourrache*; and in Middle English (from the Anglo-French), *bourage*. All of these names derive from the Latin word *borra*, meaning "rough, woolly hair," a reference to the coarse hair that covers borage leaves and stems. While an American encyclopedic dictionary states that the word *borago* may be of doubtful etymology, it also suggests that the Latin word for heart, *cor*, was changed to *bor*, and when brought together with the word *ago*, to bring, we have a name that literally means "to bring from the heart." Interestingly, the Old French word for courage, *corage,* also uses the Latin *cor,* "heart," as a metaphor for inner strength.

Another linguistic connection is to the Celtic term *barrach*, which means "a man of courage." According to Celtic lore, ancient Celtic warriors drank borage-infused wine and painted their bodies blue with the dye from its flowers as they prepared for battle in order to invoke courage from this medicinal plant. An even older name comes from the Arabic *bu ʿaraq*, meaning "source of sweat," derived from its early use in Arabic medicine as a diaphoretic, or sweat inducer. Other members of the borage family, Boraginaceae, also known as the forget-me-not family, have names that can be traced back to Arabic.

There is something truly unforgettable about borage. What sets it apart from other members of the same family is its beauty mark of prominent black anthers forming a cone in the center of the bright blue, star-shaped flower. In milder climates borage may bloom continuously for most of the year, with multiple flowers blooming simultaneously. It is a prolific, self-seeding annual herb that will appear year after year in the same patch of earth, and in the garden, borage is a bit unruly. Rough and straggling as it reaches two feet or more in height, the entire plant is covered in stiff, prickly hair. The stem is round, hollow, and very succulent. The leaves have a mildly salty taste and are rich in potassium, calcium, and mineral salts. Due to the presence of potassium nitrate, the leaves put on a light show when burned and will sparkle and pop.

The fruits, four brownish nutlets, are crushed to extract their oil. Borage gets its modern commercial value as a crop used to produce borage seed oil, one of nature's richest plant-based source of gamma-linolenic acid (GLA). GLA, an omega-6, essential polyunsaturated fatty acid, cannot be produced in our bodies and must be obtained from food sources. The essential fatty acid (EFA) in borage seed oil is used to treat inflammatory symptoms such as arthritis and chronic skin disease such as psoriasis, eczema, and acne.

The scent and delicious flavor of borage is reminiscent of cucumber as it also contains traces of the chemical compound aldehyde, an organic compound obtained by oxidation of primary alcohols. The leaves are a good source of vitamins A and C, riboflavin, niacin, and other minerals, which may explain why it has traditionally been used as a cooked green vegetable.* Fresh stems can be peeled and eaten like celery, and young leaves and flowers may be added raw to salads or infused along with mint, which makes a refreshing and restorative summer drink. Combine blue borage flowers with bright orange and yellow nasturtium blossoms to create an elegant touch to any salad or plate. The fresh blue starflowers also make a lovely cake decoration, and were candied, jellied, or made into syrup by our great-grandmothers. When dried, they add a touch of color to potpourri.

Borage flowers produce one of the only known edible blue dyes and impart color and flavor when infused in white wine vinegar. The cherished fresh, crisp flavor of borage and its medicinal qualities are enhanced when extracted in wine, and during the Middle Ages in Europe, this concoction was thought to lift the spirits. It is also speculated that borage was one of the secret herbs in the original British summer drink known as Pimm's Cup, a mixed drink containing Pimm's No. 1, an infused gin, first produced in 1823.

Borage maintains its status as a traditional cooked green in many Mediterranean cuisines. The succulent stalks and leaves have been boiled or sautéed and combined with other wild spring greens in delicious dishes like *pansotti al sugo di noci,* which is triangular pasta filled with sautéed greens and served with a creamy walnut sauce, from Liguria, Italy. It is a versatile addition to the dishes of many cultures: in Jamaica it is used with fish; in Germany, added to green frankfurter sauce; and in France, infused in cream sauce and made into soufflés and quiches.

In the kitchen garden, borage is grown not only for its herbal and culinary

---

*Borage contains pyrrolizidine alkaloids, a chemical compound that can cause liver damage in some individuals. They are the same compounds found in comfrey, only borage has 5 percent of the alkaloids that comfrey does. Long-term use (more than one or two months of daily use and internal use by anyone with a history of liver disease) should be avoided. Borage seed oil does not contain this alkaloid. Occasional use of borage as a culinary herb poses negligible risks of toxicity.

qualities, but also to discourage insects from attacking nearby plants. It is a good companion plant for tomatoes, legumes, spinach, and strawberries. The brilliance of borage flowers makes it a beautiful addition to any herb and flower garden. Borage is a green manure crop, replacing much-needed nitrogen when turned back into the soil. One of the great benefits of borage is that it is not susceptible to pests or diseases, and at the same time that it repels harmful insects, it is highly attractive to bees. While borage may be favored by beekeepers for increasing honey production, it should not be confused with the tall blue wildflowers of another plant in the Boraginaceae family, viper's bugloss (*Echium vulgare*), which is used to produce Blue Borage Honey in New Zealand.

Borage not only increases the honey production in bees, but also increases the milk supply in lactating mothers and is one of nature's best tonics for stress and the adrenals. The medicinal properties of borage can be attributed to its calming, cooling, and soothing actions. It strengthens the nervous system, regulates the hormonal system, and alleviates premenstrual and menopausal discomforts. As a diaphoretic, borage helps break a fever. As a demulcent, it reduces the symptoms of head colds, bronchitis, and respiratory infection. The mucilaginous nature of borage is soothing to both internal and external inflammations and swellings. Applied externally as a poultice, borage acts as an emollient and is beneficial for rashes and eczema. It can also be used as an eyewash or gargle.

Contemporary use of borage as a healing herb continues to evolve. It is now being drawn on as a vibrational medicine for both homeopathic and flower essence therapies. Added fairly recently to the homeopathic pharmacopeia,* borage is a specific remedy for strong-minded people who may become abrasive or angry to the point of rage when not listened to, or who may have difficulty compromising. They may also be unable to listen to others or see a different point of view. Borage-type people may often display a fear of failure and have a history of taking on the role of the parent in relationships. They may also have

---

*The principles of homeopathy require the discovery of the action of a medicinal substance through an empirical process known as proving. The evaluation of borage for homeopathic use was conducted under the supervision of Stephen Olson and published in the proving journals in 1997.

a habit of assuming too many responsibilities, resulting in resentment and a tendency to become overly protective, or even strict and authoratative. There is a sense that they must attend to every detail or a catastrophe will befall the family. Homeopathic borage brings spontaneity and playfulness to a person who has been overburdened by family responsibilities. It relieves the person's anxiety about the family's welfare, thus releasing authoritarian tendencies and the argumentativeness that stems from an overprotective nature.

Flower essences therapeutically address the mind-body connection, the emotional body, and the soul. A flower essence is a subtle liquid extract taken orally and is prepared from a sun infusion of the flower in pure water. Flowers are cut with minimal handling and dropped directly into a glass pan or jar filled with pure spring water and allowed to sit in the sun for three to five hours or until the flowers start to wilt. After the flowers are carefully removed from the water, preferably with a leaf from the same plant, an equal portion of brandy is added as a preservative. The sun infusion is then bottled and shaken for a few minutes to "fix" the remedy.

Purity, vibrancy, and celestial influences are all considered in its preparation, as the life-force energy of the plant is contained in this infusion. It is a marriage of heaven and earth. The sun penetrates the earth, and the earth gives rise to the renewing essence of the flowering plant. This energy medicine works on our subtle energy bodies and influences our mental, emotional, and physical bodies. When we turn our attention inward, we can see this as speaking metaphorically of the inner light of a Central Sun, giving rise to the essence of divine nectar that flows within each one of us. This essence contains within it a holographic imprint of the entire universe. It is big medicine.

Take this one step further and you have Earth-Spirit Medicine, in which the archetype of a particular herb, in this case borage, can interact with us at any level, and the more conscious we become of these subtle energies, the more we are able to come into relationship with the herb. Since healing takes place in the context of relationship, we are able to affect healing at the quantum level, which in turns lifts and heals all of humanity.

The borage flower essence is used specifically to help people who lack confidence in a world full of difficult challenges and is useful for those facing harsh circumstances. It restores courage to a person whose heart is burdened and conveys a certain buoyancy and lightness to the soul. It restores an individual's confidence and enthusiasm for life.

THE DIVINATION

If you have called on the medicine of courage in these troubling and transformational times, then borage is a powerful ally. As you enter the Medicine Wheel Garden and find the unruly, yet beautiful patch of blue starflowers growing between the spinach and the strawberries, know that these times are no more difficult than any other in our human history. What is different now is that we have the spiritual capacity to overcome the limits of reason. The stresses of our modern-day lifestyle are certainly taking their toll, but the physical and spiritual medicine of borage is a tonic to support and restore the adrenal glands and to bring comfort to our hearts. As we move beyond the rational mind and into the mystical realms, we find ourselves informed by a more integrated psyche, where both shadow and light are invited to dance on the stage of our life.

We are all surrounded by electromagnetic waves of energy, of which color is more than just a small part. The color blue as it expresses through these sacred flowers carries the higher vibrational frequencies that we associate with water and sky and planet Earth as seen from space. Blue is the color of spirit and of purity. In Hinduism the blue coloring of Krishna and Vishnu is symbolic of their connection to the infinite and the divine. Another Hindu deity, Hanuman, the monkey god, is seen as a source of strength and devotion. Hanuman temples are the most common public shrines in India, where one can go to receive courage in times of trouble by chanting the name of Hanuman or by singing his hymn, "Hanuman Chalisa." And while many of the stories surrounding these deities involve elaborate battles of good against evil, it is for the internal battles that we have most needed courage. But even these internal battles are ending.

It takes courage to live in the present moment, accept what is, and allow the unfolding of our life without the need to change or judge. When we can find a place of acceptance, we can move forward to create a future without fear. Engaging in battle with external forces will no longer be necessary. Borage teaches us about this kind of courage, the courage to look within, face our fears, and release them. It is a courage instilled by beauty. All the external authorities to whom we have given our personal power would not exist were it not for the promulgation of fear. What has been a masquerade of bravery in truth was a misguided sense of courage. This human experience was necessary, nevertheless, in order to learn about personal power. Marching in the face of danger promoted by authorities to whom we have externalized our power, because of a choice to live in fear, has perpetuated the fear-control-fear cycle that is now ending. As sovereign beings we no longer need to choose fear, for the biggest fear of all was of our intuitive and psychic abilities. If we think about the "borage type" as described in homeopathy, we may see the similarities of how this is expressing through a collapsing patriarchy.

As a sovereign being, you have the ability to pollinate new ideas from the flowering of like-minded people in much the same way that borage pollinates itself from different flowers on the same plant. And while the unfolding of human consciousness is happening much more rapidly than at any other point in our human evolution, not all flowers open at the same time. We would do well to embrace the beauty of all the stages of opening. The alignment of the stars is such that we are being set free to expand our view of the present situation. It takes courage to accept responsibility for what we are creating.

Borage's beautiful blue star-shaped flowers and leaves that feed our heavenly bodies are rich in nitrates that sparkle when ignited and mirror the starlike quality of our own celestial ancestry. If we take a closer look at how we have stewarded the planet with which we have been gifted, we would see that we live in a totally different world than the one we inherited. One of the ways we can take better care of ourselves, and our Earth, is by becoming aware of how we are in relationship to the elementals. While nitrates are an essential source of nitrogen for plants, nitrogen-rich fertilizers used to enrich soils eventually leach into the groundwater, causing contamination. This contamination has led to a potentially fatal blood disorder in infants under six months of age called blue baby syndrome.* This disease is not required to

---

*Human infants have bacteria in their digestive systems that convert nitrate to nitrite, a toxic substance. Methemoglobinemia results when nitrites are absorbed into the blood, decreasing the oxygen-carrying capacity of hemoglobin in babies and potentially leading to death. The Environmental Protection Agency (EPA) has set a maximum contaminant level for nitrates in drinking water, and levels above this are known to cause this potentially fatal blood disorder.

be reported by doctors or laboratories in some American states, or in other countries where water quality is threatened, and it is often mistaken for other illnesses, making it difficult to determine the true incidence of blue baby syndrome, even though a simple blood test is conclusive. Research also suggests that exposure to high levels of nitrates may cause cancer. There is no simple or reliable way to remove nitrates from drinking water.

This is important not only because of the widespread use of highly concentrated nitrogen fertilizers (either chemical or natural) that can potentially contaminate drinking water, but also because of the incidence of mothers who are not breastfeeding their infants until at least six months of age. Blue baby syndrome is the result of mothers feeding babies infant formula made with well water containing high levels of nitrates. This is compounded by the fact that bottle-fed babies start eating solids many months before breast-fed babies, who usually start wanting solids around six months of age, and vegetables fed to bottle-fed babies contain naturally occurring nitrates, adding to the load. The digestive system is not equipped to deal with solid food before six months of age, let alone nitrates. Many doctors believe that blue baby syndrome is much more widespread than statistics indicate.

When Marcel Vogel explored energy medicine in the 1970s, he discovered that the energetic patterns of a fertilizing agent could be stored in a crystal and then transferred into water. He found that when this water was used to irrigate plants, they showed a significant growth increase compared with untreated plants. Perhaps we could allow the purity of borage's little blue star-shaped flowers to remind us that all of nature is exquisite in its beauty and perfection. In learning to create a dialogue with nature, we can find powerful alternative solutions to the problems we are currently collectively facing. To face everything that you create with courage is one of the lessons of borage.

Borage also teaches us to remember who we are. This plant was born in the cradle of civilization, an area known as the Fertile Crescent, and reminds us that we have been starseeded. We know that a seed cannot grow without first lying in still, cold darkness and that nothing will flower without the warmth and light of the sun. As we learn to be gardeners of the heart, we will emerge from the darkness and be warmed by the light of a Central Sun as our souls take flight. The New Testament story about Paul on the road to Damascus takes place in the area where borage was starseeded. The story speaks of spontaneous illumination and revelation about oneself. It is also a metaphor for bringing cultures together. We are currently at such a boundary of change, as evidenced by the instability of our borders, which are simply arbitrarily drawn lines separating people, countries, religions, and states. The age of separation is ending as the age of illumination is dawning. On the road to Damascus we may discover borage growing by the roadside as we learn the truth about who we really are and where we came from. This sudden turning point in our evolution allows us to see both sides of the story of good and evil as we integrate them into a new worldview and old belief systems fall away. We stand in a portal of great change at the turning of the ages and have been gifted with a great teacher and ally in the starflower we call borage, who seems to be saying, "Take heart and have courage."

Gazing, soft-eyed, through the silvery cast of this white-haired elder, into the clear blue stars of this medicinal plant, something ethereal starts to emerge. This five-pointed blue star has been a powerful image through the millennia, representing religious and political systems of belief and prophecy, as well as healing systems across the world. It is heralded again in our times as we call on the courage to face the difficult times ahead without being discouraged or overcome by fear. Drink deeply of the divine nectar of starflower's essence and receive the courage that will lead you into your greatest joy, as together we birth a New Earth.

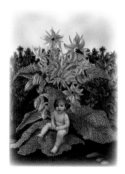

THE DEVA SPEAKS

My medicine is Star Medicine from the Blue Star Nation of the Sirius constellation. I have informed the building of your pyramids and am brighter than your own sun. Both are lighting your pathway home to the Central Sun. You have been receiving my radio waves of transmission for eons. Put down your cell phones and pay attention! It's time for us to have direct communication. The plants and planets are electromagnetic beings just as you are, and that is why they have influenced you. It is time to reawaken to the importance of the heavens. Each star impulses you. Call forth your own light and broadcast your own transmission, for this is your time. It takes courage to walk into the sun.

I will share with you a simple secret for activating your life-force energy: Lie naked in the sun. Take the sun as your lover, and feel the heat within you rise. The sun star is a gateway through which you must pass in order to become one with the spirit. This is the intimacy that humanity has been longing for, this union with the sun and the activation of your kundalini. For many it lies dormant, like seeds beneath the soil. Waiting. Waiting for just the right amount of moisture. Look at your life right now. Is it moist? Are you warm and warmed by the love of all that surrounds you? For all that surrounds you *is* love. The sun gives rise to life, quickens, inclines, and reaches its zenith, and then declines as it sets back into the earth so that conception, incubation, and rebirth may continue. Every day is a new life. Each life is birthed new with each new day. Become alive. Marry with your sun and give rise to the masculine within you. Fall in love with the moon and make love to the stars. Know the incredible human being that you are.

I am here to restore courage to your heart and remind you of the star that you are. The stories of bravery among you are many, but the stories of true courage are few. Courage can live only as long as love is in your heart and on your tongue. All victories lie with the vibration of love. And what of those who gave their lives in the name of service to humanity? What would they say to you now from the other side? They would say they died for a cause. They died to set you free, and still you battle for freedom.

Beneath the shield of the Cheyenne warrior, you are given strength. Yours is the heart of courage residing in the heart of Hanuman. When you are willing to give all that you are and all that you have to become whole and healed, then all that you do will become sacred. When all that you do becomes sacred, you will become whole and healed. Yours is the courage to dream a future not yet in form.

Allow me to assist with your understanding as you learn to interpret the sacred mysteries. When you take the understanding into your heart that all of life is sacred, that everything is holy, then everything on Earth will shift to a higher frequency. You have the potential to create a utopian society from this knowledge.

Those of you who are committed to healing on a multidimensional star path will find yourselves pursuing many different interests—careers, hobbies, and relationships—for how else would you develop all the facets of yourself that are curious and inspired to explore the workings of the universe? It takes courage to pursue many different interests when you may never get good at any of them. Since you were not guided from childhood to follow your passions and interests, but were groomed for productivity and success as determined by your parents, teachers, and culture, you never really got to taste the fullness of a passionate life unfettered by the expectations of others.

History has proven that free thinkers are persecuted. This memory is carried in your DNA. You have been sold many truths, but the truth cannot be bought or sold, and the time has come to shift your perception beyond what you think. As you move into your hearts and unleash the love that is within you, previously shrouded in fear, you will find that you have the courage to both speak and live your truth. Use my medicine to reconnect your heart with the source of the divine that lives within you.

You are both creators and destroyers by the laws that bind you to your dimension of duality; you have been gifted to explore these polarities, and you have done well at both. Your ability to destroy life on this beautiful green planet is extraordinary, and so is your creative ability to touch the heart with a profound beauty. And this beauty will endure. Not here in this dimension as you know it, but beyond anything that can you can imagine. You are encouraged to imagine. It takes courage to dream.

If you find yourself standing on the shore of a sea of broken dreams, when a way of life is ending and someone you love leaves, never to return, know that it takes courage to face what will remain. What have you lost and what will you gain? While you know that there is no going back, why do you hold so little hope for the future? Perhaps it is a future that cannot sustain your insatiable desires and greed. I ask you to look within and know that you will always have everything you need. The universe unceasingly sustains you. This is the moment when you gather all your courage and take the next evolutionary step of faith. Whatever form it takes. I bring you the physical and spiritual medicine of courage and the Star Medicine of transformation. With my stars to guide you and my medicine to heal you, you will find the courage to take one whole heart home. Yours is the courage to love, the courage to heal, and the courage to leap.

Until the heart opens with courage the temple door is barred.
The muse waits for the strong heart, to give the right mind.

BHAGAVAD GITA

I am yesterday and tomorrow, and have the power to regenerate myself . . . the hitherto closed door is thrust open and the radiance in my heart hath made it enduring. I can walk in my new immortal body . . . and go to the domain of the starry Gods. Now I can speak in accents to which they listen and my language is that of the star Sirius.

THE BOOK OF THE DEAD
(ANCIENT EGYPTIAN FUNERARY TEXT)

Blessing of a Star

I wake in a world of darkness,
these days before the dawn,
and lift my eyes to sunrise,
and the blessing of a star,
for we are all born of stars,
as night falls into day,
and day falls into night,
as night falls into stars.

I stand bare and naked,
before leafless trees the same,
their silent branches praying
for a blessing of the rain.
In darkness no rain is falling;
the air is quiet and still;

still I hear a quiet voice
beyond my windowsill.
It speaks to me in visions;
it tells me where you are;
it teaches me to know
the blessing of a star.

I dance in a circle,
birthing, things tender, new, and green;
there lies the promise
of a blessing for the spring.

Leaves turn brown and golden now,
as daylight turns to dusk,
and night falls all around us,
as night falls into stars.
In a circle ever turning,
where breath is song enough,
the river holds the secrets of
a ruby in the rough,
and the promise of a future is not so very far
from the source of love within us
or the blessing of a star,
for love it is that moves us;
it tells me where you are;
it teaches me to know
the blessing of a star.

THEA SUMMER DEER

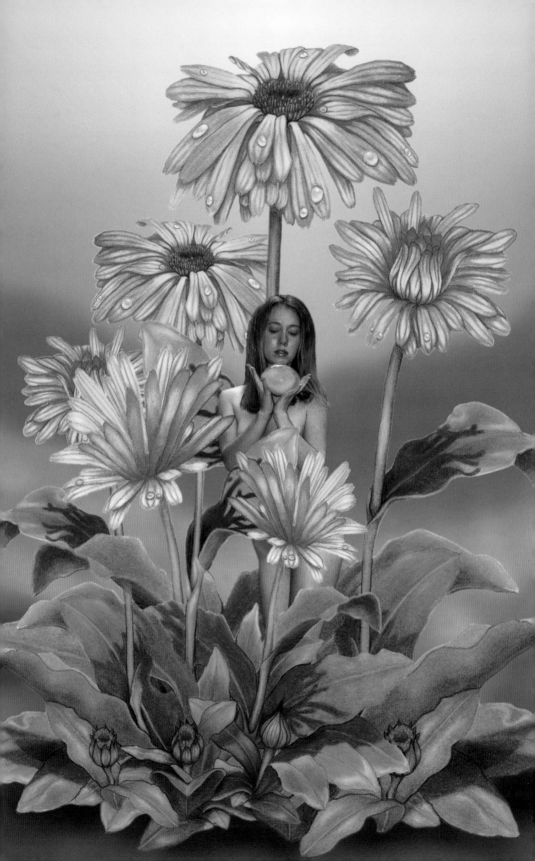

Calendula

Calendula officinalis

Subtlety

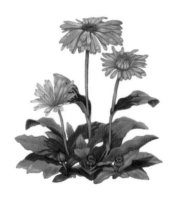

Bright and beautiful *Calendula officinalis* derives its name from the Medieval Latin *calendae,* which means "day of the new moon." This was also the first day of the month in ancient lunar calendars and refers to the plant's tendency to be found blooming throughout most of the calendar year. The botanical Latin word *officinalis* is an adjective meaning "used in medicine." In the Western European herbal tradition, plants that carry the species name of *officinalis* have some of the oldest known therapeutic uses in the herbal pharmacy, or materia medica. Calendula is certainly one of our oldest and best-known allies.

Calendula is more commonly known as pot marigold in Europe, but it is not a true marigold, whose genus is *Tagetes*. Calendula and marigold both, however, are members of the Asteraceae family, formerly known as Compositae. This is the daisy family, which includes the sunflowers, and it is the largest family of flowering plants, rivaled only by the (mostly) tropical Orchidaceae family. The Asteraceae, despite their simple appearance, are

45

highly evolved plants containing separate male (disk) and female (ray) flowers on the same plant.

The early Romans brought calendula, a native of North Africa, back to Europe from Egypt. Highly prized by both the Egyptians and the Romans, calendula was also known and used by East Indian, Arabic, and Greek cultures. Because of its long history of cultivation and the ability to self propagate, it is naturalized in temperate zones throughout the world.

Calendula is an annual that grows one to two feet in height and width. It grows best in well drained, rich, but somewhat sandy soil, and prefers full sun. Exceptionally hardy, it can grow in both acidic and alkaline soils and in semishaded areas, and while it requires moist soil, it doesn't tolerate being overly wet. It is easy to germinate, selfsowing, and blooms quickly after sowing, usually around a month.

The Old Saxon name *ymbglidegold,* meaning "turns round with the sun," describes calendula's sensitivity to light and temperature. Its flowers open in the morning, follow the sun's light during the day, and then close at dusk or when it is clouded over. Calendula's ray flowers express themselves in shades from creamy yellow to brilliant orange and deep orange reds. Flowering from spring into fall, calendula bears light green, lance-shaped leaves, which give off a distinctive exotic odor when crushed, as do the flowers. It is commonly grown as an ornamental and makes a very attractive border plant. Wildlife also finds it attractive, as do its pollinators: bees, butterflies, and hoverflies, which eat aphids. Calendula is a good companion plant in the garden for this reason and is normally free of pests and resistant to disease.

While there are many species of the genus *Calendula,* only *C. officinalis* flowers are used medicinally or as an edible. Its traditional use in the cooking pot is more than likely what inspired its name of pot marigold, rather than the containers in which it may be grown. The golden petals can be used as a spice to add color and a subtle, yet distinctive flavor reminiscent of saffron to cooked dishes. Sometimes called poor man's saffron, or Egyptian saffron, it is similarly employed as a yellow dye for fabrics, cheese, and cosmetics. It can also be used fresh in salads and as a colorful and decorative garnish. The leaves may also be added to salads but tend to be somewhat bitter.

As a healing herb, calendula has been used medicinally in a multitude of preparations and is one of the most versatile herbs in Western herbal medicine. Its soothing nature and anti-inflammatory properties make it suitable for internal and external use. Preparations include cream, ointment, carrier oil, and infusion, applied with a compress for external use. Internally it can be taken as an extract, an infusion, a powder contained in capsules, or a tea. Depending on the preparation, calendula may be used to treat pain, bleeding, acne, and skin and mucous membrane inflammations, and to promote wound healing. It can be applied topically to cancerous tumors and used to prevent infection. Calendula's healing properties soothe stomach ulcers, bedsores, rashes, sore throats, gingivitis, and other conditions of the mucous membranes of the mouth. It is useful as an eyewash and for the treatment of varicose veins. Used throughout Europe as a heart tonic, it also has a positive effect on the liver, with its bitter principle aiding the secretion of bile.

Additional internal applications include uses for fevers and jaundice. Many mothers know the value of calendula as a safe and effective diaper ointment. Truly a woman's friend, it can be used to soothe sore or cracked nipples, to stimulate delayed menses, and to treat vaginal yeast infections. The herbal actions of calendula are many, and it has been suggested in plant pharmacological studies that calendula may be protective against substances that are known to be potentially cancer causing or capable of causing genetic mutation, and that it may have antitumor (cytotoxic) activity. These are important considerations on our current evolutionary journey.

With as many gifts as this plant has to give to humanity, it is no wonder that it has been considered magical. Certainly the synergy involved in its ability to heal is greater than the sum of its constituents. According to the Doctrine of Signatures, an early method of identifying the healing properties of plants based on their appearance or the environment in which they grew, calendula was observed as being both sad and cheery. Dew droplets, which collected in the flowers during the night, were seen as tears of grieving, perhaps for the loss of her love, the sun. As the first rays of her returning beloved shine on her face, drops like tears fall from her petals as she opens to receive him. Calendula's dance with the light and the dark has inspired many a poet, including Shakespeare, who was moved to write, "The marigold, that goes to bed wi' the sun, and with him rises weeping."[1] This endows calendula with yet another common name, the poet's marigold.

Christians have long associated marigold, the gold of Mary, with the Virgin Mary and in the seventeenth century with Queen Mary. While these associations may seem like religious or political opportunism, a more subtle connection may link calendula, the flower of grief, with Mary Magdalene. First consider that Mary Magdalene's other name was Maudlin (excessively, tearfully sentimental) and that she was a follower of Jesus (the Sun of Righteousness). Then taking into consideration that the Old French word *mariée*, meaning "spouse" or "bride," is used in the word *marigold*, another name for calendula, a picture emerges of how this healing plant may connect Magdalene with Jesus as the bride of the sun. Another flower in the Asteraceae family, *Chrysanthemum leucanthemum*, whose common name is maudlin daisy, provides yet another link to calendula's association with Mary Magdalene.

THE DIVINATION

In the early morning of a new day, when the dew is fresh on the ground, enter the Medicine Wheel Garden, where the flower of gladness and grief is found. And when you find yourself in the presence of calendula, know that her bright and cheery nature will comfort you in your grief. Whatever you have perceived as a loss, lay calendula on the altar of your grieving, in the temple of your heart, and receive a healing and rejuvenation of the spirit.

The world is only just now waking up to the truth of who Mary Magdalene was as a high priestess, not a whore, and the sacred union she shared with Jeshua. Much was lost in the fall of Magdalene. Not only did the world lose a body of sacred knowledge when this and other truths were denounced as false doctrine, but also the teachings of sacred marriage and of our connection to the divine. We lost the subtlety of meaning in our lives. With this subtle shift in perception and the way we began to think and feel about ourselves, we lost a whole navigation system. Dominated by linear thinking and oppressed by patriarchal control, we stopped taking our cues from the subtleties of nature. While this was a necessary stage in our evolution, we are now entering a new phase of understanding.

As we open at this time to a new world, a new dawning at the shift of the ages, let us also open to the increasing light on our planet. This light comes from the solar flares of our own sun star and from the increasing illumination of consciousness. As the old is burned away and we grieve the loss of what has come before, the dream of a new day is unfolding. Call on the spirit of the Magdalene high priestess to assist you at this time. Her legacy is one of endurance through the dark night of the soul and the ability to perennially bloom.

Learn to read the subtle signs of prophesy and the changing winds of time. Learn to dream and to remember your dreams. Messages are waiting there for you. The communication that you seek is within your own soul. When we learn the language of the soul, our misunderstandings evaporate in the light of a new understanding, one that allows us to have compassion for all sentient beings. True compassion results from embracing both the dark and the light within you, and in others.

Calendula is most certainly one of our wise old elders, and while her closing at night may be a metaphor for grief, her opening speaks of joy. At this point of paradox we find the truth of our Higher Selves, which is a rhythmic dance of shadow and light. When you allow this gilded flower to speak to your heart, the illusion of separateness dissolves. As one species gives rise to another in a spiral dance of interdependence, we find that we are not separate from all that is, that we are interconnected. The language of science sheds new light on this ancient understanding. When we learn how to be in compassion, we create a bridge to a new expression of humanity. Subtle as these feelings and intentions may appear, they generate new connections: to the earth, to ourselves, and to each other. How we think and feel about ourselves sets up a sympathetic resonance that touches all of creation. From this resonance a New Human Being is emerging. This is the song of a New Earth, where we rediscover what it means to be truly human and to live in harmony.

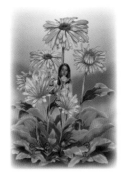

THE DEVA SPEAKS

So you would ask of me, "How is it that you have come to teach us of subtlety, when you are one so radiantly full of color and light?" And I will respond by asking you to look within and see how far you have come from that which is closest to you. You are radiant beings beginning to remember the subtle truth of who you really are. *Know yourself,* because what you are becoming is dependent on your integration of who you presently are.

These are your last hours of ancient sunlight. There was a time before your sun was created, and there will be a time after it is destroyed. There are many more suns than there are incarnate hearts. Your spirit will travel on to other worlds, and in fact your journey is only just beginning.

You will feel shards of light exploding in your body, and this is an experience that I know intimately as a light being. It was during one such explosion that our bodies were created anew and we emerged from the sea. And so it is for you now at this time of transformation; your bodies are becoming something more, something new, something filled with light.

The physical body that you now inhabit is vibrating within the geometric pattern of a six-pointed star. Yours is an inner technology that resonates with the higher frequencies of the universe. Your ancient ones called this vehicle a Merkabah. Through this vehicle you will be transported to the next dimension of manifestation and time.

Followers of the sun, you have become confused in your devotions. What is within you is infinitely subtler than the object of your senses. And in fact you are now discovering the many more senses that are within you, many more ways of perceiving an even greater world than the one you presently inhabit. These senses have lain dormant within you, waiting for this time, for this new beginning when you turn your face to the Central Sun of your being and become the flower of life that you were born to be. Blossom and sow the seeds of a greater consciousness, for a greater humanity is seeking expression through you.

You are male and female within the one, just as I am before you. Do not judge the sexual explorations of your kin. It is through this exploration that you will discover new parts of yourselves in each other. It is necessary for your evolution. Practices that are not sustainable to your species will fall away; it is the Law of Nature. Let yourselves be guided, drawn to the light that calls you, and all of your expressions will become sacred.

Focus now on your breathing; it is an exercise in subtlety. Subtlety is what opens the heart. Ah, but if you knew that in your courting, how much more successful might you be! For truly you have been courting power, but this power has eluded you in its subtlety.

Listen now to this message of the heart: remember the subtle power of the rhythm of light in your bodies. What is subtle are your female bleeding cycles called forth, as are the changing tides, by the moon. Your footsteps fall in rhythm with the turning of the seasons, or in due course, carve out the rut of your existence in a linear path that you traverse daily. These mysteries are the domain of the Goddess, whose gold is a treasure that lies within you, and you have always been its source. When you find out what you have, you will stop measuring your life by what you don't have. Precious metals and gemstones ripped from the body of your mother lie much more subtly in the heart of your inner knowing. Use them where they lie. It is not necessary to mine them outside of yourselves, for what value are they once removed? Rejoice in the value of your own inner sourcing, for you are priceless beings, each one of you a star in the constellation of humanity. What was stolen from the Goddess was done so very subtly over a long period of time. It is the gold that runs in my veins. As you rediscover this endless treasure within yourselves, I too am healed and become the queen of a New World.

Your true gold shines within you and is a reflection of your own Central Sun. These things are subtle, and you are robbed of them daily by your attention to the chaos and clutter. The color of my disks and rays is but a reminder that you are at the center of your own solar system.

Subtlety is relative. What was previously perceived as subtle becomes gross the finer tuned one's perceptions become. Those who do not choose to become conscious are becoming denser, more fragmented. When we no longer open to the light, we fade back into the elementals from which we are made. There is no right or wrong choice. Ice has more density than steam. Snowflakes are uniquely individual fragments of the same element. When a Central Sun warms you, your consciousness perceives light at higher vibratory levels. I am here to remind you to face that light, bow reverently to the darkness, weep for what has been lost, and rejoice in the coming of a New Age.

Calendula's Beloved Dance with the Sun

Subtly she turns
Slowly at first
Greeting the warmth of her lover's true light

Subtly she opens
Spreading her rays
Waking from the darkness of her soul's longest
*   night*

Open to receive all that's been given
A new day is dawning; the old one has ended

Subtly she waits
Collecting the kiss
Of a lover who knows how to touch her like this

Subtly she closes
Her day is done
She surrenders herself to the breath of the One

Open to the morning's first rays of light
Closing herself to the darkness of night

In the glorious rays of the sun she will bask
And the golden threads of her petals give back
For in all of the gifts that a new day will bring
He is her Lord and she is his Queen

THEA SUMMER DEER

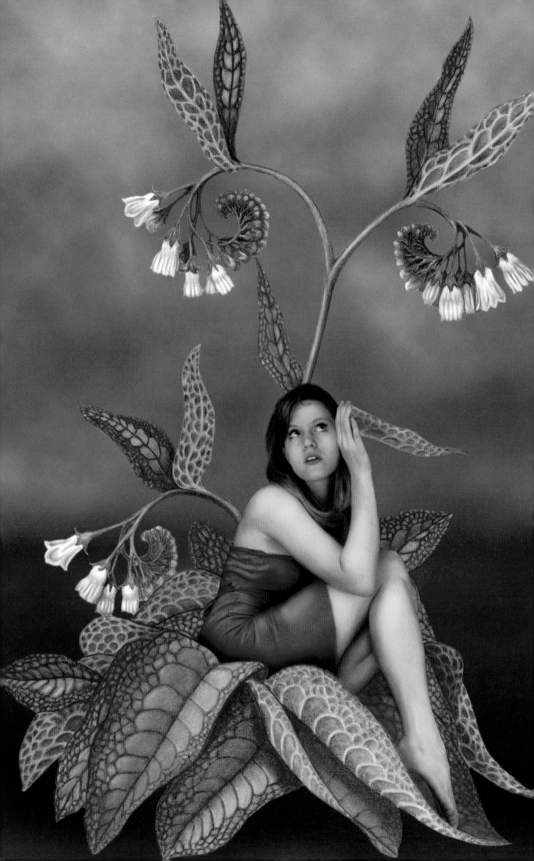

Comfrey

Symphytum officinale
....
Healing

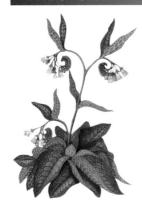

The botanical we know as comfrey, *Symphytum offi-cinale,* is a miraculous plant that long has been used to heal damaged skin and mend broken bones. Both the common and botanical names reflect its healing actions: *Symphytum* from the Greek word *symphyo,* "to grow together," and comfrey from the Latin *con-firmare,* "to unite or to heal." In olden days another common name for comfrey was knitwort. The suffix *-wort* on the common names of plants gives insight into their traditional uses. According to the *Oxford English Dictionary, wort,* or the Old English *wyrt,* is an archaic name for a healing plant, root, or herb.

The prefix indicated the ailment or complaint for which it is used. Knitwort is a plant that knits tissue. The term *wort-cunning* was used to describe someone who was skilled in using roots and herbs for healing. After the seventeenth century, the word fell out of common usage. However, the name *knitwort* may still invoke an ancient memory for those of European descent whose ancestors used this herb in healing.

Comfrey is native to northern Europe and, along with borage, is in the

Boraginaceae family. It is a hardy perennial with thick roots, and it grows approximately two to three feet in height. The basal leaves are large, six to fourteen inches in length, and covered in rough, prickly hair. In some species, contact with leaves may cause irritation and itching. The deep green leaves decrease in size the higher up the stem they grow, terminating in racemes of pale blue, bell-shaped flowers. Like other members of the Boraginaceae family, comfrey flowers grow only on one side of the flower raceme. As the flowers bloom from May to August, the tightly curled stem unfurls from the bottom to the top, each flower blooming one at a time as the raceme eventually straightens. This type of flower arrangement is described as "scorpoid," as it resembles the curved shape of a scorpion's tail. The flowers are bisexual, and in species that produce seed, the fruit consists of four shiny nutlets.

Comfrey encompasses a symphony of species. Cross-pollination of these species has resulted in a range of flower colors, from white and blue to pink and even yellow. As a result, it has become increasingly difficult to differentiate between species. Botanists believe that common comfrey is descended from two parent species, European comfrey (*S. officinale*), with white or pale blue flowers, and prickly comfrey (*S. asperum*), with blue flowers and native to the Caucasus Mountains and western Asia. The species most commonly cultivated is *Symphytum uplandica,* a hybrid cross of these two parents with darker blue or purple flowers, also known as Russian comfrey.

Russian comfrey is far more widespread than either of its wild parents and was widely cultivated in Europe as a source of livestock feed. It is a hybrid that never sets seeds and propagates itself through root proliferation and cuttings. Joseph Busch, who was the head gardener at the palace of Catherine the Great at St. Petersburg in Russia, originally introduced Russian comfrey to English gardens in the late 1700s, where it was grown as an ornamental. Busch fell in love with the healing powers of comfrey and sent roots back to his native England from Russia for cultivation.

Another hybrid is *S. peregrinum*. English farmer and Quaker Henry Doubleday propagated this species in the mid-1800s, which he used successfully as both food and medicine in livestock applications. Doubleday, the inventor of postage stamp glue, was searching for an alternative to gum arabic when he began to investigate the mucilaginous nature of comfrey. The Henry Doubleday

Research Association was founded in England as a result of his explorations. The original comfrey roots used by Doubleday in his experiments were also taken from the gardens at the palace of Catherine the Great in Russia.

Continuing Doubleday's research in the 1900s, Lawrence D. Hills became the director of the Henry Doubleday Research Association and is credited as the father of organic gardening in the United Kingdom. Hills worked with comfrey extensively and wrote the book *Comfrey Past, Present and Future* in the 1950s. His work with comfrey included measuring yields, disease resistance, and the composition of various cultivars. He discovered that one particular hybrid, which he named Bocking 14 after his hometown, along with an assigned number, produced a yield of almost forty tons per acre.

Comfrey is a welcome addition to any organic garden. It likes rich, moist soil and prefers full sun, but will grow almost anywhere. Most often started from root cuttings, comfrey is drought tolerant due to its deep taproot, which can reach as much as six feet in depth. This long root also allows comfrey to absorb nutrients usually only taken up by tree roots; it draws potassium from the soil, making it an excellent soil amendment, especially useful for tomatoes. When used as mulch fertilizer or to activate garden compost, the leaves decompose rapidly, releasing nitrogen and enriching the soil.

Herbalists have used comfrey for more than two thousand years. Dioscorides, a Greek physician, first documented comfrey's use, as a vulnerary to treat wounds for the army of Alexander the Great. A common plant found growing in damp soil and alongside ditches in much of northern Europe, it was a popular remedy in the Middle Ages, when it was frequently used as a poultice. The mucilaginous roots were grated and mixed with water to form a kind of plaster, which was applied to broken bones and fractures. While it was the preferred "bonesetter" by these herbalists, comfrey doesn't actually set a broken bone, but once the bone is set, comfrey's ability to reduce swelling and stimulate tissue growth speeds the healing process.

Two important active ingredients of comfrey roots are mucilage and allantoin. Some research indicates that the roots may contain 8 to 10 percent allantoin, a chemical constituent also found to a lesser degree in the leaves and flowers. When a preparation of comfrey is applied to the skin as a poultice or salve, the allantoin is easily absorbed through the skin, where it promotes cell growth to speed wound healing, reduce scarring, and soothe irritation and inflammation. Comfrey also heals mucus membranes and is especially useful in healing perineal tears and abrasions or an episiotomy following childbirth. An infusion of comfrey leaf combined with a decoction of the root, used in a warm sitz bath or applied as a hot compress, ensures a speedy recovery of this area. Comfrey also softens, moisturizes, and protects the skin against irritants, making it an essential ingredient in salves and ointments for the treatment of wounds, burns, bruises, cuts, sprains, sunburn, chapped lips, cold sores, diaper rash, and skin irritations. Wounds, however, should be cleaned thoroughly, as comfrey may cause the surface skin to heal over first, potentially trapping infection. It is not recommended for deep puncture-type wounds for this reason.

Comfrey is largely grown and used as animal fodder. While studies to determine comfrey's toxicity have been done primarily on rats, numerous studies show the benefits of using comfrey leaf as an animal food supplement, especially for cattle, since it contains two essential amino acids, lysine and alanine, which are missing from alfalfa, a common animal feed.[1] Allantoin is also considered important for the maintenance of digestive system health in cattle.

The internal use of comfrey for people is controversial, even though comfrey tea was traditionally used in Western herbalism to treat digestive system irritation, sore throat, and coughs, and it was eaten as a nourishing food. Recent advancements in our understanding of phytochemistry have resulted in recommendations to restrict its internal use.

Although it is rich in nutrients, including calcium, chromium, fiber, manganese, potassium, protein, selenium, silicon, amino acids, and vitamins A, B, and C, comfrey also contains chemical constituents known as pyrrolizidine alkaloids (PAs). PAs exert their toxicity by destroying liver cells or causing abnormal cellular growth that can lead to severe liver damage or even cancer. The variability of PA content from one comfrey plant to the next presents a challenge in assessing its risk. U.S. Food and Drug Administration (FDA) studies show extreme variability in the PA content of commercial comfrey products, and as a result, their sale is restricted.* While both the leaves and roots are used

*The American Herbal Products Association issued a policy that all commercial comfrey products sold by AHPA members should contain the warning that the product is intended for external use only and that it should not be used by nursing mothers nor applied to abraded skin.

medicinally, alcohol tinctures of comfrey are not advisable, as alkaloids extract well in alcohol. It is best to restrict comfrey use to oil and water preparations for external use only. It may be wise for people who have had any form of hepatitis, chemotherapy, alcohol abuse, or liver disease to avoid comfrey altogether.

The debate over comfrey's potential toxicity to humans illustrates an important political issue: that of government regulation and control of herbal supplements under the guise of consumer safety. Unfortunately, the regulatory process often relies on the opinions of those who have never given herbs to patients: researchers, manufacturers, bureaucrats, and academics. Statistics support the fact that most exposure to poisons does not involve plants. In contrast, the statistics on poisoning and death from conventional drugs and pharmaceuticals is staggering.

Whenever government control of a substance is introduced in an effort to save consumers from themselves, we are given the opportunity to look at an even deeper issue, the one of personal responsibility in health care. Certainly accurate information should be made widely and easily accessible so that informed choices can be made, but the general lack of a consistent, efficient regulatory system for medicinal plants in the United States has hampered consumers and health care providers from obtaining knowledge of the potential dangers of certain plants. In the following quote, published in the *New York Times*, we can see the root of the problem in our current health care system. The system supports victims and heroes, and the problem is one of *not* taking personal responsibility. "The lack of quality standards is the No. 1 problem in the whole industry," says Dr. Varro Tyler, professor emeritus of pharmacognosy (the study of medicines derived from natural sources) at Purdue University. "I feel sorry for the typical consumer. How is he or she to know what is best, what products are reliable and safe?"[2]

Paradoxically, the money it would take to accurately evaluate the safety and effectiveness of herbal products would necessitate the involvement of government and pharmaceutical companies. This would certainly alter the regulatory and political climate surrounding medicinal herbs, further controlling and limiting, not expanding, our choices in health care. The illusion is that this kind of regulation would make herbal medicine legitimate. What it actually does is take away our individual responsibility and control what is available, both in terms of products and education. The pharmaceutical companies already control the dissemination of knowledge in our medical universities and in the private practice world of doctors, who are wined and dined in exchange for hearing about how to push the latest drug.

We have taken health care so far out of the hands of the people that we have become completely dependent on someone outside of ourselves telling us what is safe. We have lost not only a whole navigation system, but also the continuity of life itself. The more we allow the regulation and control of our food and our medicine, the more we lose control over our individual choices and personal freedoms. Empowered with information and good models for health and healing, people will make empowered choices. If we choose to continue to allow ourselves to be robbed of these choices because we fear the processes of life and death, we will lose that which is essential to being human—free will and sovereignty.

THE DIVINATION

If you have entered the Medicine Wheel Garden in search of healing, then you will find it here, where the deeply rooted comfrey grows. She is a perennial healer who knows the cycles of darkness and light through the changing of the seasons, and she comes back every spring to offer her healing once again. In this same manner, we die and are reborn throughout this lifetime and many others, returning to receive the healing of a new season. We have literally walked lifetimes through harmony and discord, and through seasons of health and vitality, contrasted against a backdrop of sickness and dis-ease. It *is* possible to be well all the days of our lives. This potential once was and still is a reality. Though we may still get "sick," because that is why we have developed an immune system, it doesn't mean that we have to suffer. Suffering is the result of resisting rather than surrendering to our higher guidance. We have the tools to transcend suffering if we are willing to take the time to uncover them from their long slumber of disuse.

Planted within us are seeds that hold the potential for healing. These tools are not given to us by someone else; they already exist inside of us. This potential for healing is realized when the seeds are warmed by the light of love and what the devas call a Central Sun. Only then do these seeds grow into the medicines that heal us on every level. During this time of tremendous transformation, some of which may bring illness to our bodies, minds, and spirits as we adjust to the shifting frequencies, we are challenged to remember the restorative power of the cycle of the seasons. A death cycle is one such adjustment that is restorative and is not to be feared, fought, or denied.

Human suffering is a paradox. Some of our greatest healers and shamans have received their initiations through illness. Saint Teresa of Ávila (1515–1582) is but one example of long suffering endured in order to bring forth a great teaching about the human condition in relationship to a higher power. The list of martyrs, saints, saviors, and shamans who have brought us this teaching is extensive, but what they have all tried to tell us and show by their example is that we can rise above suffering. If we listen carefully we may actually hear them say that they suffered so we wouldn't have to. On the other side of suffering is healing.

Some believe that comfrey can cause suffering in the form of physical damage when taken internally. Some believe that comfrey is a great healer when taken internally. Beyond the story of science and belief is an energetic frequency still waiting to be discovered. Comfrey is a spiritual medicine that does not require ingestion. This plant is capable of healing through the vibration of sound, but you have to slow down if you want to hear it. Depending on where you are standing in the Medicine Wheel Garden, comfrey is striking a chord, a series of notes that are resonating in harmonic frequency with the vibrational pattern of the current stage of your life. This plant sings us awake. If you take time to meditate in the Medicine Wheel Garden and comfrey appears to you, listen to her message. It is meant for your personal healing, and ultimately for planetary healing as well.

Healing is something that happens when you step into the frequency that supports the resonance of life, of which death is a part. Some call this frequency *love*. The root of comfrey, which reaches deep into the earth, draws up elemental energies in the form of minerals and crystals. Comfrey's bell-shaped flowers ring the harmonic truth that when we heal in this lifetime, we heal those who have come before us and those who are yet to come. When you tune in to these elemental frequencies, you are listening to the messages of your ancestors, for we all have evolved from the second dimension of the elementals. They *are* our ancestors.

If you allow comfrey to become your ally, you will find that you have the support you need to be transported to a place where all is whole and healed. The third dimension that expresses in matter will always know the duality of sickness and health; it is the law. It is not our job to change it but to accept and integrate it so that we can move toward healing and ultimately on to other worlds and dimensions. It is our sacred purpose. Many healers are already accessing other dimensions through the vibration of sound. It is no longer a matter of visualizing a world that is whole and healed, although this has been an important exercise, but a matter of *knowing* that a reality where we are whole and healed already exists and is not something to be achieved. As this world of possibilities becomes known to us, we pull it into our consciousness from what might appear to be the future, but what is actually happening is a softening of vision that dissolves the boundaries between past, present, and future and opens a more expansive view.

We are wired for wholeness. If you think about people who have been "healed" from cancer or some other life-threatening disease, one of the things that they have in common is they have made some kind of major change in their lives, possibly a change in career, marriage partner, or where they live. In other words, they died to their life as they knew it, so they didn't have to die altogether. Another way of looking at how we are wired for wholeness is the example of when someone loses a limb, possibly an arm or a leg, and stills feel an itch, tingle, or sense of movement in that limb. This is how our brains are electrically wired for wholeness. This is also true for a woman who has lost her ovaries or uterus but still feels the twinges of ovulation, or for a woman who changes her menstrual cycle to match the phase of the moon or another cycling woman in close proximity.

A place exists, not just in our brains but also in the dimension from which our very form is created, that is wired for, and remembers, wholeness. It is the place where our spirit lives before we take on a physical body and to which our form returns. And while these are examples of how we are *physically* wired for wholeness, we are *spiritually* wired in a similar manner. We can achieve spiritual healing through a kind of soul retrieval in which our soul re-members all the other parts of itself into wholeness. It is the space and time where we remember ourselves as being one with all that is. We are still learning how to transcend space and time, but we do not need to die in our current physical incarnation to have this direct experience of unity. Our physical body is also wired to remember our spiritual body. We can experience oneness or wholeness while we are still in a physical form, just as comfrey experiences her deva. Many techniques are available to help us achieve this, but spending time in nature and listening to our own inner guidance and that of the devas is simple to achieve. Integrating the whole of our self with All That Is brings us the healing we seek.

One of the healing stories from our distant past that illustrates this truth tells of Egypt's Isis and Osiris, who are metaphors for life and death. In this tale, Isis, the embodiment of spirit in flesh, dances with the death of her beloved, Osiris, as he lies in the underworld like a seed beneath the earth. Osiris's journey into death and dismemberment is essential in order for new life to be reconstructed and for the journey to continue. It is also the story of subconscious truths rising to the conscious mind and of the past and future merging in the present.

What is born of this death, dismemberment, re-membering, and rebirth is something wholly new, and in this case it is Horus, the new king. It is the birth of a new consciousness. And when one chooses to die consciously, whether to life as we currently know it or to this incarnation altogether, the resurrection that ensues is the birth of the future in the present moment. This birth is the hope and healing of all generations, past, present, and future. It is where the whole of who we are is able to respond to the whole of who we have become and are becoming. It is where illness and suffering become an opportunity to reawaken. Through all the songs and stories of our past, comfrey sings to us from our future to awaken in our ever-present now. As Isis awakens Osiris from his underworld sleep and he rises up to meet her, our consciousness too rises up to create new forms, new bodies, and a New Earth.

Comfrey teaches us that healing, knitting together what has been torn apart, is not a linear process but a spiral journey. Millennia of indoctrination have taught us well about the linear path of cause and effect. We have spent many years on our evolutionary journey reasoning our way through illness and looking for its causes. In the most recent of these years, we have explored the possibility that our thoughts might be making us sick, but you can't have a debate with illness. Neither is an illness something that comes and lands on you, and poof, you are sick. Multidimensional healing cannot be approached from the limitation of the mind. The mind is the servant of the ego, not of the higher dimensional self. When the mind is surrendered and focused on holy breath, the crown chakra is opened to divine guidance, and the root chakra is anchored to the timeless center of the earth, when these polarities merge through the love we are capable of holding in our hearts, then we are transported into the ether, where we can witness the creation of form as one might watch an artist painting a masterpiece.

To think that a "negative" thought could be the cause of an illness is a reductionist mode of thinking that is self-perpetuating. We heal when we get out of our minds and vibrate at the frequency of love. Healing takes place in the context of relationship, and we are all related to All That Is. Negative thinking, or any other kind of destructive or self-destructive behavior, does not exist within a frequency of love. Healing in this context is not about curing symptoms or removing negative blocks, but about healing our lives. It is not about going to a healer, but about becoming our own healer. Comfrey so loves the ground in which she grows that she holds open a door for us, a green healing door, into the deeper truths of who we really are. And while it may be an old cliché, love *is* the greatest healer. Touché! No one goes untouched by love.

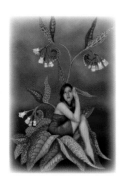

THE DEVA SPEAKS

Dearest ones who seek to heal and be healed, my medicine is your gift. It is a tool with which to clear your bodies and your minds. The emotional body is the last explored frontier of your human self and psyche, and without a clear body-mind you cannot access the pure emotions that are your navigation system to a new dimension. My gift to you is this: pass one of my roots over your body in much the same way that you would pass a crystal. This will ground the chaotic energy that leads to your imbalances and dis-ease. After you have grounded your energy, you may then pass my root, from head to toe, over someone who is experiencing an illness. This will pull the sickness down and through the body and into the earth, where it can then be neutralized. As long as you are living and swirling within chaotic and ungrounded energies, you are "spinning out," as you like to say, and are distracted from the essence of who you truly are. Listen as I sing you back to center, as I bring you back to the center of the garden. For it is here in this sacred garden that you will find my harmonizing medicine to heal you.

It wasn't that long ago when you became aware that in order to heal, you must heal on all levels: physical, spiritual, emotional, and psychological. But now you are expanding into levels of multidimensional healing. It is important that you have the ability to feel into yourselves through a clear emotional body. When you heal in the present moment, you change the events of the past and shift the probability of the future. You are healing now at the quantum level with the aid of my spiritual medicine. When you hear and receive my song, we heal each other. When you heal, I heal.

My leaves and flowers heal your conscious mind without your ever needing to take them into your body, and my roots heal your subconscious without your even needing to dig them up. I will knit you back together when you embrace me for the whole of who I am. When you come into harmony with all of the facets of your multidimensional self, you will know what is needed, and at what time and in what amounts. Use my roots to stay grounded and my leaves and flowers to stay centered.

As you heal on a physical level, look for the Medicine Men and Women who are not afraid to use unconventional means. Medicine Women are the keepers of the medicine roots, and they know how to use and apply this kind of healing energy. It has taken many years of practice to learn how to use this strong medicine. These healers are quick to act in a healing crisis, and panic is not part of their sacred medicine. Many healers are among you now, and they have learned how to use power without forcing the energy or exerting their will over another. It is the animal nature within you that has fought aggressively for your healing and created the aggressive healer. This was necessary for your healing and survival in the past. I am here to tell you that it is no longer necessary for you to fight for what you want or believe, but it *is* time to stand firmly grounded in the knowledge that what you need is already fulfilled. It is time for you to understand the difference between yourselves as conscious human beings who have free will and as the animal that must survive. For what would you survive?

I will tell you the story of my brethren and of my ancestors before me. For eons we have been tuning ourselves to the music of the stars. I, the lone sister, rode the starway of light to your beautiful blue green Earth, impulsed by the elementals, who at the time were creating great works of form and color but had not the music with which to animate their creations. I came at their beckoning, bringing with me my brothers, whose voices were rich and deep. Together they sounded the heartbeat of our Mother Earth. So penetrating were their voices that she conceived her song and gave birth to me in my current comforting form. I am the embodiment of light and sound. And because the Mother's heart beats true and my brothers' love for her is deep, and because I heard and answered the call, traveling on wings at light speed, my love for all of my Mother's creations has kept me tuning and retuning, checking and rechecking the frequencies of creation in the symphony of life. This is the moment we have all been waiting for. All of the rehearsals, the deaths and rebirths, this is the moment when the music is perfected and the first chord is struck. Feel its power, for it is a symphony of heavenly bodies beyond your brightest imagination. You are magnificent beings who are not only alive at the turning of the ages, but alive with sacred purpose.

Healing is not what you think. It is a mystery discovered only by those who walk its path. Healing is never accomplished alone or in isolation. It is a dynamic force that is activated within all your relationships. It is a resonance in which all that is discordant is brought into harmony with all of the other parts. When you not only see, but know, that our Mother Earth is in her pristine, pure, flowing essence of form, for indeed she is, and when you see the organs of your body as vital and functioning, for indeed they are, then you will know that dis-ease is transient and wholeness is eternal. When you choose to heal on any level, it is an act of power. Your resonance, your note, your chord that is vibrating in this symphony of life is an essential part of the song of a New Earth.

Comfrey's Multiverse

Lift me up
into your hands of clay;
sing to me
your song of days,

and I will sing
to you my song of night,
shifting now
in the ever-changing light.

Earth magic
lifts up to you, my friend;
deep dark earth
holds healing medicine,

from my heart
feel the sound increase,
as I impart
the grounding that you seek.

THEA SUMMER DEER

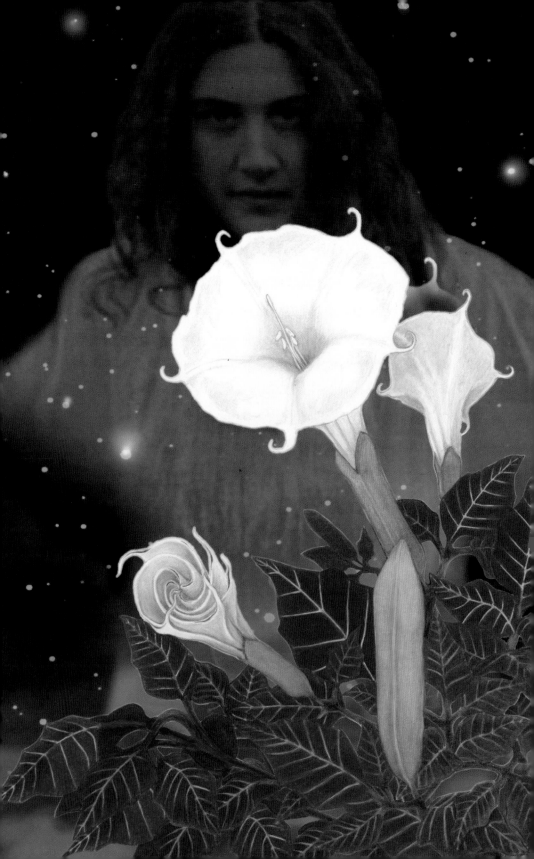

Sacred Datura

Datura wrightii

Night Bloomer

THE STORY

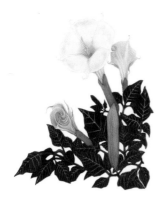

Sacred datura (*Datura wrightii*), also known simply as datura, has a long history of shamanic and ceremonial use and was considered blessed by the Indians of Mexico and the American West and Southwest. It belongs to the Solanaceae family, also called the deadly nightshade family, which includes several potentially toxic members, including tobacco, belladonna, mandrake, and henbane. Paradoxically, this family also includes such common food plants as tomato, pepper, potato, and eggplant. Its night-blooming flower is an intoxicating, lovely, large white blossom, commonly referred to as moonflower, not to be confused with the cactus night-blooming cereus. Although its association with night and the moon aligns it with the feminine, sacred datura has been attributed with both feminine and masculine traits by the cultures that used it. To the Aztecs, datura was *toloatzin* in their native Nahuatl tongue, a male plant of the gods. To the Chumash Indians of south-central California, it was *momoy,* a "powerful old woman." Momoy, a Contrary* gave birth to Coyote, the trickster and sorcerer. To the Spanish, datura was *yerba del diablo,* "the devil's weed," or more commonly, "locoweed." In many parts of Mexico, the plant was known as *toloache* and used in divination and vision quests to seek a spirit helper.

The genus name *Datura* is derived from the Sanskrit *dhatturah,* translated as "thorn apple," an accurate description of its distinctive thorny fruit. Dhatturah appears in the ancient Vedic scriptures, which were gathered together in approximately 1500 to 1000 BCE, but are thought by some to be much older, perhaps written five thousand years ago. The species name, *wrightii,* commemorates the American botanist Charles Wright. During his long botanical career, Wright collected plants for Asa Gray, one of the most important American botanists of the nineteenth century. Wright was a great explorer, and his expeditions into Mexico with the United States and Mexican Boundary Survey resulted in collections that led to this species name honoring his work.

Datura consists of fifteen species, and all contain similar properties. The species that most likely originated in South Asia is *Datura stramonium^* which closely resembles *D. wrightii,* and both are often referred to by the common name jimsonweed. Today, jimsonweed can be found all over North America as a roadside weed. *D. stramonium* is one of the fifty "fundamental" herbs in Chinese medicine, a system of medicine that recognizes the interconnectedness of life and uses herbal remedies to bring the body back into harmony with the universe. Stramonium, a homeopathic remedy prepared from this species, is used to treat Parkinson's disease and night terrors in children. In India, datura has been used to treat everything from malaria, heart disorders, and earache to impotency and baldness. It can also be used to relieve painful engorgement of the breasts by placing two to three applications of warmed datura leaves on the breasts.

Sacred datura is a vigorous herbaceous perennial that grows up to five feet tall. It is a striking ornamental with sweet, fragrant, white trumpet flowers that open after dark and wither at sunrise. Spiny walnut-size seed-

---

*A Contrary is a shaman who takes a stand in opposition to the current state of affairs with her own contrary power in a complementary dance that is a play of power.

pods split when ripe to release numerous seeds. The longevity of these seeds may be responsible for sacred datura's success as a weed. The symmetrical corolla has five parts that are sometimes tinged with purple at the margins. Sacred datura is pollinated by hawk moths. These moths are large, the size of a hummingbird, and are sometimes referred to as sphinx moths because when they are in the caterpillar stage, they assume a sphinx-like pose when frightened. Sacred datura is also a larval plant for some Lepidoptera caterpillars.

Long before the Spanish conquest, the Aztecs used sacred datura as a medicine by applying poultices to wounds to reduce pain. Aztec priests considered the seeds sacred and kept them in secret boxes on their altars.[1] The dried leaves were smoked as a bronchodilator to relieve symptoms of asthma. Asthma was not recognized as an inflammatory disease until the 1960s, and at that time, anti-inflammatory medications started to be used. Prior to that, herbal smoke inhalation was considered an effective remedy for potentially life-threatening asthma, and herbal inhalation remedies were used as far back as ancient Egypt. The Ebers Papyrus, found in Egypt in the 1870s by Georg Ebers, contains prescriptions for these remedies written in hieroglyphs.

In Hinduism, Lord Shiva was believed to have smoked datura, and his devotees still leave an offering of the thorny fruit on the Shiva temple altar. Datura is referred to in ancient East Indian literature as *shivashekhera** because of the believed association of Shiva with datura flowers.[2] Shiva is a somewhat paradoxical god, with both masculine and feminine attributes, as well as the reputation as both destroyer and benefactor, fearsome and benevolent. The five-petal corolla of datura may correspond to the sacred number that is associated with Shiva. For example, there are five mantras for Shiva, the most important one being *Namah Sivaya,* which contains five syllables. The image of Lord Shiva has inspired generations of painters, and datura flowers are often depicted in Hindu Tantric art.

One of the most beautifully inspired modern depictions of sacred datura may be Georgia O'Keefe's painting titled *Datura and Pedernal,*

Shekhera is an epithet of the Hindu god Shiva and means crest or crown.

which depicts a floating datura flower in front of Pedernal Mountain in New Mexico. The beauty, inspiration, and healing of this plant is in stark contrast to its power to bring death and destruction. Romanticized in legends, ceremonies, myths, literature, and art, sacred datura's reoccurring theme of beauty and danger make it an intriguing plant.

Beyond the danger and the intrigue is the very real story of the experimental uses of sacred datura. One of the plant's active ingredients is scopolamine, and it is classified as a deliriant. The delirium that it produces has been likened to a psychotic break, in which subjects are delusional with minimal control over their actions and little to no recall of the experience. Not fully comprehending the spirit of this plant, scientists created the drug scopolamine from deadly nightshade's alkaloids. The dark nature of this drug was exalted in the 1950s, when it was used in combination with morphine and administered to women in labor to induce "twilight sleep." Women who requested it or whose doctor prescribed it for them would take it during the throes of labor in order to give birth without the memory of pain. It caused the mother to be completely removed from the birth experience and gravely depressed the baby's central nervous system. Twilight sleep was once much sought as an alternative to pain in childbirth, but it remains a dark chapter in the history of obstetrics.

The main alkaloids in datura are atropine, hyoscyamine, and hyoscine, also commonly known as the daturine alkaloids. These alkaloids cause paralysis of the eye muscles and affect the nervous system, with atropine acting as a stimulant and hyoscine as a depressant. A more promising modern use of deadly nightshade includes bioremediation, in which the alkaloids absorb heavy metals polluting the soil.[3] Soil contamination by TNT and related explosives is a problem at military installations in the western and southwestern United States, where datura grows abundantly.[4] Bioremediation is of particular value in the removal of TNT. The alkaloid hyoscine in sacred datura has also been identified as an antipoison remedy for organophosphate, nerve gas, and puffer fish exposure.*

---

*The Tetraodontidae family, which includes puffer fish, contains at least 121 species in twenty genera. *Takifugu rubripes* is the most highly prized edible species and the most poisonous, containing the neurotoxin tetrodotoxin. It is believed to be the second-most poisonous vertebrate in the world. When the Japanese delicacy *fugu*, made from puffer fish, is not prepared properly (most commonly by uncertified handlers), poisoning occurs.

Sacred datura is a power plant that has both creative and destructive aspects to its personality. Its internal use has never been considered pleasant and can cause a complete and violent break with reality and even death. Sacred datura ingested even in small doses can be fatal, and for this reason it was used to commune with the spirits of the dead. In parts of South America, indigenous peoples used sacred datura to induce intoxication and deaden the senses of women and slaves before being buried alive with their dead husbands or masters. Prior to the 1800s, it was used by the Chumash in puberty rites ceremonies in which a boy returning from his ritual intoxication would forget who his mother was. This made him no longer a boy who belonged to his mother, but a man who belonged to the tribe.

The Algonquin Indians of Virginia practiced a similar rite. Other uses include divination to find lost objects and shamanic journeying. The latter is surprising, because under sacred datura's influence, the break with reality is so complete that one does not remember the visions it may have induced. Humankind has used sacred datura since time immemorial as a poison, medicine, and ritual intoxicant, and as a means for acquiring personal power.

THE DIVINATION

At the edge of the Medicine Wheel Garden, just beyond the low wall that separates darkness from light, you will discover the sacred moonflower of datura. If you pause long enough and wait for the dying sun to set, her scent will lure you to come closer. As light fades to dark and you find yourself standing in the presence of this sacred medicine plant, be cautious, or you may find yourself courting a disastrous break from reality. If you have forgotten who you are and where you came from, datura will remind you of the areas of your life in which you are not being present. Many souls are fragmented and lost at this time, searching but not knowing or finding that for which they search.

Sacred datura has the ability to erase memory, and you will not be able to re-member yourself or discover the answers to your soul-searching until you step out of the reigning darkness. She may seduce you with promises of personal power that lead you into the desert at night, but if you choose to follow her, your lessons will be difficult and you may not remember them when and if you do return. She is a master of illusion. The illusion is that it is safer to open toward the darkness than to open toward the light. You may not have felt safe enough to open toward the light. But even sacred datura knows how to open to the light of the moon, a reflection of the sun's true light.

If you are dancing with sacred datura as she is dancing with you, it is time to wake from your twilight sleep and immediately go into the dark and painful places inside of you where you have watered the night-blooming flower of darkness. Your trauma has caused a kind of amnesia, and you have forgotten the places where your soul fragments lie. The further you fragment, the further you descend into the world of sacred datura. Her medicine serves as a reminder to bring back what is lost. Until you bring these pieces back, this powerful old woman will trick you into thinking that your illusion is reality. You may have convinced everyone around you that you are functioning just fine when in fact you are giving your essence to the night.

So many lost souls are searching today for any kind of personal power they can find in a world that leaves them feeling disempowered and disillusioned. Many search through the medicine plants, which they abuse as they have been abused. Honor the sacred medicine of datura by discovering the flower in you, which in spite of the violence and abuse still blossoms in the darkness beneath the only light where she feels safe. Sacred datura mirrors the beauty of the flower that you are, just as the moon reflects the light of our solar sun.

When you step out of the darkness, you will feel and know that you stand in the light of something much greater. You may have been living in a bad dream, but it is time to replace the hallucination with a vision. Those who repeatedly call on the medicine of sacred datura tend to live in isolation and lose their ability to discern reality. If this sounds like you, then it is time to ask for help. If you are making the soul retrieval journey or are traveling through the dark night of the soul and the sacred world of datura, it would be advisable to seek a shaman or "one who sees in the dark." Some medicines are best left to the initiated.

We hold in cellular memory everything that has ever happened to us. Sacred datura has the ability to erase these memories or remind us to retrieve them. If memory is erased, what then will take its place? She serves as a Contrary, as a shaman who teaches us about the play of power between two opposites that are part of the same whole. When we stand in darkness and are opposed to the light, we are in essence serving the light in its opposition to darkness. When we embrace her, we lose the fear that keeps us in the darkness. The darkness is seductive and could show up in your life in myriad ways, from addictions to self-destructive behaviors. Repressed traumas may be responsible for an undeveloped psyche, which may be unable to discern the danger of sacred datura. Sometimes we study what we don't want in order to understand what it is that we do. When you discover the flower of sacred datura that blooms in the darkness inside of you, admire the beauty of her existence, her history, and her evolution, and then leave her to her world as you return to yours. You cannot bring the flower back with you, for it will perish. When you remember what has been lost, you can retrieve it, but once you retrieve it, you should release it. Learn how to forgive, and you will ultimately forget the pain from your past.

Once a memory has been released, it may be surprising how easy it is to forget the circumstances that created it. It's similar to the way we forgot where we came from when we descended into physical reality. When we retrieve our lost soul parts and release the associated memories, the pain will fade as we move into the light, fade until it is long forgotten and nothing but a dark chapter in the history of our collective human consciousness. And even these memories will fade on the day when we wake and discover that we have been made wholly new *en una nueva tierra*.

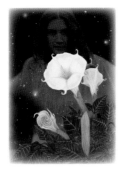

THE DEVA SPEAKS

Datura, do you remember where you came from?

No, I have erased all memory of the past.

If you don't remember where you came from, then how can you know where you are going?

Deva of my flowering essence, I do not need to know where I am going, because the future is not yet in form.

But how can you have a future if you do not have a past?

Because of you, my dear deva, the memory of my evolution is kept safe so that I may create the illusion of power that lies in violence and knows only darkness.

Is it true, datura, that those who follow you by ingesting your flowers, leaves, or seeds will also know only darkness?

Yes, it is true, but you, my precious deva, hold the distant memory of starlight, which is reflected in the light of the moon. It is in this light, the place of all beginnings and endings, beyond the memories of time, that I bathe my flowering essence. It is this light that my followers seek.

If those who seek your medicine embrace you for who you are—a flower that lifts her face to the light of the moon—and they don't try to take you back into the light of day, will they remember where their lost and broken soul pieces lie?

Those who choose to embrace me for who I am will be guided in how to bring the pieces of their fragmented souls back into the light of the living, leaving me to flower in my darkness. I teach through contradiction; I flower in the darkness, but I am in deep harmony with the day; I am life that is in harmony with death; I am earth in harmony with sky; I am what is seen and what is unseen; and while I am real, I dance in the illusion. They acquire my true power by listening to your wisdom, the wisdom of the deva, not by following the illusion.

Thank you, datura, for allowing me to serve you so that you may transcend the memories of this time and bring a great teaching to all humankind.

The lady of moth and moon unfurls her shy and deadly petals. These navigators of the midnight sea—occultists and poets and devotees seeking after that which seduces them—are familiar with the dream of intoxication that follows her scent. She is the woman in the song, the night-blooming narcotic, gorgeous and strange. She is the horned blossom, the guardian of the threshold, the keeper of madness.

RUBY SARA

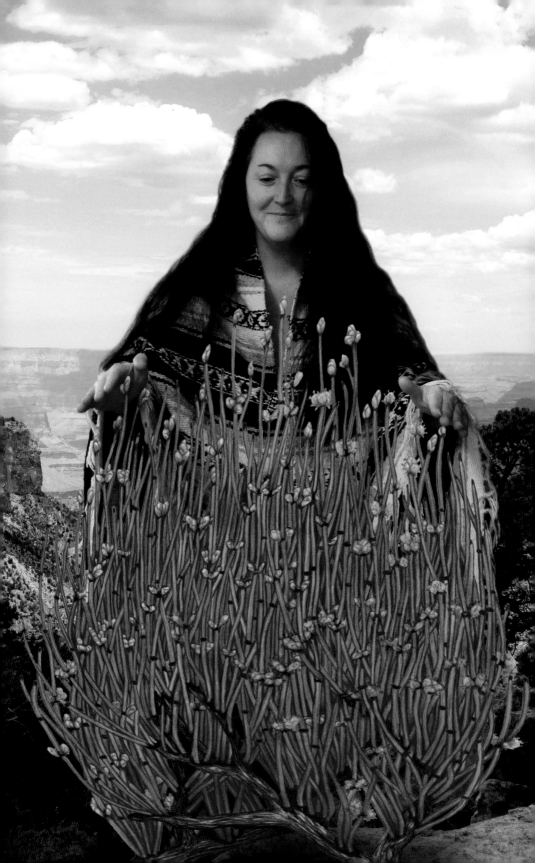

Ephedra

Ephedra viridis

Anchoring

THE STORY

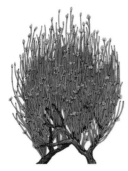

The Mormon tea family, Ephedraceae, has but one genus, *Ephedra.* The species found extensively in the Great Basin region of the United States is *Ephedra viridis,* whose common names include Mormon tea, joint-fir, and green ephedra. This easily recognizable, erect, evergreen, broomlike shrub is drought resistant and winter hardy. It typically grows waist high but has been reported growing up to six feet. Ephedra has a slow growth rate, with most of its growth occurring in the cooler months and needing full sun. It is found rooted in rock and sand, sharing the same habitat as creosote bush, sagebrush, saltbush, and Indian rice grass. The deep roots of ephedra act as an anchor to stabilize sandy soil and help prevent erosion in the desert. Ephedra, with its vivid green color, stands out among the monotone colors of the desert landscape.

Ephedra is derived from the Greek words *epi* and *hedros,* which mean "sitting upon." The word has its origins in the genus name for horsetail, *Equisetum,* which it resembles. The species name, *viridis,* is Latin for green.

Approximately forty species of ephedra exist worldwide, and five species live in the Four Corners region of the United States. *Ephedra viridis* is the most common variety found growing on the mesas and in the canyons of this region. It is also abundant in western Texas and in the mountainous deserts and foothills of southern Central California. It is an important plant in the ecosystem and plays a major role in restoring and rehabilitating western rangeland communities and other disturbed areas because it reduces erosion, reestablishes quickly after fire, and helps reclaim land damaged by mining.

Ephedra is one of the oldest and most primitive plants on the planet. It is a nonflowering gymnosperm, or naked-seeded plant, like pine, juniper, and spruce, and it has a taste and smell reminiscent of pine. Its leaves resemble tiny, dark scales and are incapable of photosynthesis, which instead takes place in the green stems. The male and female spore-producing cones are wind pollinated and located at the joint or node of the needle, with the male featuring prominent yellow pollen sacs. The seeds have a sweet, pleasant, licorice-like flavor, and they can be ground and added to flour. Deer and cattle graze on ephedra plants, while quail and deer mice eat the seeds. The nutritional value is fairly high, making it an important winter food source for these animals. However, ephedra is highly toxic to domestic sheep and cows during gestation, but surprisingly not at other times.

When disturbed, ephedra may spread by producing new sprouts from the roots. Small mammals that use ephedra for ground cover also aid in dispersing its seeds, which may be viable for over a decade. It has been observed that the male plants grow on dry windy spots, while the female plants, which require more moisture, are found in wetter areas. Ephedra grows at elevations up to ten thousand feet and can survive with less than ten inches of annual precipitation.

Other common names given to ephedra by early European settlers include Brigham tea, squaw tea, and desert tea. Mexican, Spanish, and Indian names are popotilla, tuttumpin, tutupivi, canatilla, and teposote. Hopi, Navajo, Ute, and Paiute people all used ephedra as a medicinal herb. Tea is brewed from the twigs of the plant, and the Navajos boiled the twigs with alum to produce a light brown color used to dye wool. The common name Mormon tea was probably given due to ephedra's popularity as a black tea substitute with early Mormon settlers, as their religion dictated that they abstain from caffeine.

Mormon tea may also refer to another species, *Ephedra nevadensis*, a better-tasting herb found throughout the same region. Long before Mormons claimed the herb for their tea, native peoples of Central America and the southwestern regions of North America were using ephedra to create beverages.

E. viridis is sometimes confused with another species of ephedra, *Ephedra sinica*, or ma-huang, an important herb in traditional Chinese medicine. Ma-huang is mentioned in the classic first-century-CE book *Shen Nong Ben Cao Jing* (*Shen Nong's Herbal*), the basis for the modern Chinese materia medica. This powerful plant medicine is highly regarded in Chinese herbology. *E. sinica* contains the alkaloids ephedrine and pseudoephedrine, which the pharmaceutical companies have synthesized for use in many drugs. Ephedrine is a very strong central nervous system stimulant. Pseudoephedrine is a bronchial dilator and an ingredient in many over-the-counter and prescription drugs. It is used to treat symptoms of respiratory and other pulmonary ailments, including, but not limited to, asthma, hay fever, allergies, bronchitis, coughs, colds and flu, arthritis, fluid retention, and congestive heart disease. In addition to its action as a bronchodilator, *E. sinica* speeds up metabolism and is often used in weight-loss formulas.

Pseudoephedrine is a synthetically produced drug that mimics the effect of the hormone epinephrine (adrenaline) and is similar in chemical structure to the amphetamines. This has made it a sought-after chemical precursor in the illicit manufacture of methamphetamine. The United States House of Representatives passed the Combat Methamphetamine Epidemic Act in late 2005 as an amendment to the Patriot Act, and it was signed into law in 2006. The federal statute lists stringent requirements for merchants selling any product that contains pseudoephedrine.

Ephedra, as with so many of the medicine plants, is a perfect example of what medical science is just beginning to recognize and what herbalists have always known: plant synergy. When using the whole plant (stem and leaf), all of the chemical constituents are present, balancing, supporting, and buffering each other, and no undesirable side effects have been reported. The species used by the Indian tribes of the Southwest contain little or no ephedrine.

There is a legend about the Hopi in Arizona and the Tibetans in Tibet, two very spiritually based cultures. This story tells how the two are connected through the center of the earth and have the ability to travel back and forth through an interior tunnel. Geographically they are on the exact opposite sides of the earth from each other. It has even been observed that many of their customs are similar, and the women even wear their hair in a similar style, like a butterfly. While Chinese and North American ephedras have different active constituents, there is something very powerful about their connection to each other from opposite sides of the globe. For this reason, it is the genus *Ephedra* and not the individual species that now becomes our focus.

THE DIVINATION

If you have wandered into the desert searching for a way to quench your thirst and for the strength to continue on your journey, look no further. In these times of shifting sand, ephedra's deep roots will provide you with a spiritual anchor so you may continue to explore the canyons of your soul. A spiritual anchor does not chain you to old traditions, bind you to the past, or commit you to a narrow path. The anchoring of ephedra stabilizes the shifting sand beneath your feet while the winds of change are blowing. It also allows your body and consciousness to absorb more light so that you may become more present in the unfolding plan for Earth and humanity. Anchoring connects you with where you are right now in time, unlike grounding, which connects the physical body in space through the chakras to a larger planetary grid of the earth. Anchoring is a way of sending a luminous root into present time so that our spirits do not wander and become lost. Anchoring focuses our attention in a way that allows us to observe more fully.

Anchors can also be stimulating, and ephedra models this for us as both an anchor and a stimulant. A response to a stimulus in one of the senses may also stimulate a response in one or more of the other senses. For example, a red or green traffic light stimulates us to stop and start at the right time. Anchors provide a way for the unconscious to process stimuli, much the way plants send roots into the earth and receive nourishment. With awareness we can replace unproductive anchors with spiritual anchors that root us to our soul's wisdom and bring us into alignment with our divine purpose.

The only reason that we abuse or become addicted to any substance is because we have lost the connection with our own divinity. A belief system anchored in illusion only takes us further into the illusion. Since the anchor root carries our perceptions and beliefs with it into present time, it also draws up the nourishment we need for our souls to evolve into the future and renews our connection with a deeper spiritual source. As we allow ourselves this nourishment, our perception becomes anchored in a truth that no longer chains us to a limited belief system. The practice of allowing all things creates just such an anchor, letting us walk a path of greater service.

Once we have learned how to create a spiritual anchor in our life with the assistance of ephedra, an amazing thing happens. Our boundaries change and may even disappear as the shifting sands blow across the landscape of our lives. Boundary setting was an important practice while we were still learning about our personal power. We have learned well that time and space do indeed have boundaries. But we are at a point in our evolution where these boundaries no longer serve us, and in fact, they limit our perception. Boundaries create separation and are arbitrary constructs when in truth we are unlimited beings. When we become anchored in present time through all of the dimensions, the healthy boundaries we have worked to achieve are set in place automatically without our even needing to think about them. It no longer becomes necessary for the ego to protect the little self when one is in alignment with the Higher Self. What was previously defined and defended as a boundary dissolves and becomes spiritual protection when one is spiritually anchored.

The deva of ephedra serves as a protector through its action of anchoring us in the spiritual. Healthy boundary setting in this context takes on a quality similar to that of an autonomic response. Once we become anchored, nothing can come into our field on any level that is not in service to the highest good. However, we must nurture and nourish our nervous systems in order to be able to hold these new frequencies. Ephedra's medicine is the calibration that is needed at this time.

In our present day and age, many of us are walking around exhausted from adrenal burnout and overstimulation. We have forgotten that we have everything we need at any given moment and have burned ourselves out crossing an endless desert in search of the objects of our desires. Our roots have been sent into ground that neither sustains nor nurtures. Never before has the stress on our bodies, minds, emotions, and spirits been greater. Everything we have constructed—from our cities, homes, and businesses right down to our families and individual lives—has been built on shifting sand. The winds of change are upon us. Connect yourself deeply through the spirit of ephedra, quench your thirst, and find the energy to continue your journey so that you may come home to the Medicine Wheel Garden. As you hold and drink of ephedra, allow yourself to anchor in a deeper spiritual knowledge.

One of the reasons we incarnated is because we wanted to collect the parts of ourselves that were anchored here in the past. By anchoring in the present, the dividing lines between past and future merge, and all that you have been or ever will be is realized. This is what it means to be self-realized. Know that the greatest truth of all lives in the present moment and is right inside of you. Ephedra is a medicine plant that has lived long on the earth and is in service to the winds of change that are blowing us ever closer to the moment when a New Earth unfolds.

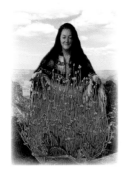

THE DEVA SPEAKS

You have crossed the fathomless spaces through impos-ing landscapes, following only your faith, but faith was never meant to be followed. Determined to practice this following of faith, you have sailed across oceans, forged the mightiest rivers, crossed the deepest and wildest canyons, built homes, irrigation systems, dams, and trails, and now you stand at the edge of something so great that your mind cannot imagine crossing it. Your faith will be replaced by the knowing that comes from anchoring in a greater spiritual truth—the truth that everything you need is always at hand and that you are magnificent beyond what you have previously imagined. You stand at the edge as One-With-All That Is. You have seen yourselves as pioneers, immigrants, explorers, prospectors, and traders, but in truth you have always stood at the edge of this Great Divide. Only now is your DNA ready to receive the instructions on how to proceed into unknown territory where none will suffer as a result of your exploration and where the sharing of knowledge will lift up the many so that not even a few will be left behind.

I am not troubled by the abuses of my medicine, for the evolution of your consciousness has needed me in the forms that your imagination conceived. As you awaken to your magnificence, where we are no longer separate, you will be able to use my medicine in its whole and perfect form, and together we will cross over into the New World. I will always be here to quench your thirst. It is through your breath that you will find my anchor. Drink and breathe deeply of me. I am the oldest of plants and have walked with you from the beginning across burning deserts and into the canyons of light. The heat that I can give you because I have risen from the deserts of the world is in support of your immune system, which is collapsing from environmental stress. My heat is anchored in the intent of the Creator; I heal you by stimulating your immune system so that it can meet the challenges you face at this time. It is not coincidental that my alkaloids mimic adrenaline. I have held this day of your need in my memory. Anchoring it in the present *is* my medicine and my gift to you so that you may continue toward an unknown future.

Blessed is this time of transition and all that it shall bring. Know that the light you seek is already within you, expanding into its fullness in the infinite here and now, anchoring you as an incarnate soul in the greatest adventure of all. I am not a being of many words, having spent so many years alone. This was necessary so that I could anchor the energies without distraction in preparation for this time. And now, at last, you have approached me for the whole of my medicine. At last you have learned how to use it wisely. I have met others at the end of their long journeys. I am a very old soul, hardy and well adapted to the harsh conditions of this world. But this is not the world that you will inherit, for the old world is passing away. I am creating an anchor for you in yet another bright green reality should you choose to follow me to the edge. It is a reality where you discover the warmth of a new sun and a new world. It is where you turn the last corner and with great wonderment and awe are the first to view the birth a New Earth.

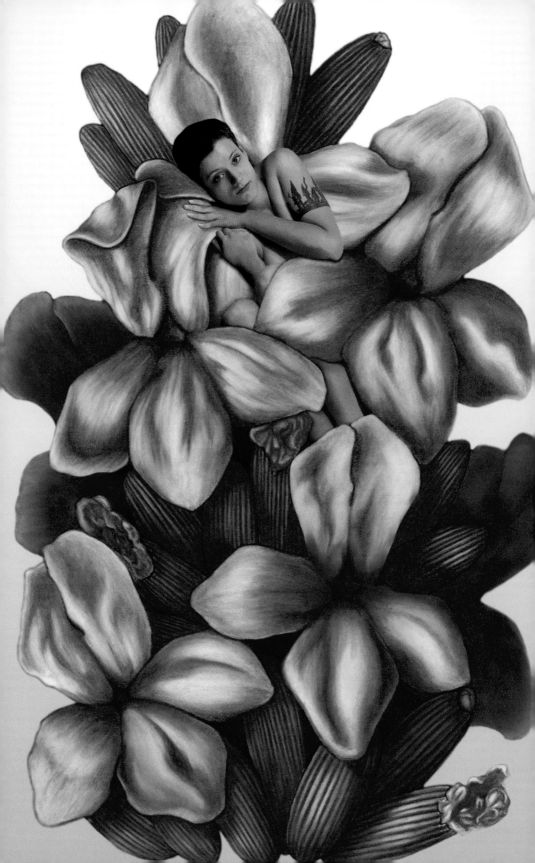

Lavender

Lavandula angustifolia
· · · · · · · · · · ·
Duality

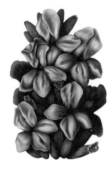

Born into the mint family, Lamiaceae, lavender is indigenous to the mountainous regions bordering the western half of the Mediterranean and extending across the Canary Islands, Africa, Arabia, and India. *Lavandula* is an Old World genus of flowering herbaceous plants with over thirty species. Lavender flowers are bisexual and cross-pollinate easily, resulting in an abundance of variations within the species. Lavender buds and flower spikes, both fresh and dried, are used in the fragrance, specialty food, entertainment and tourism, and alternative medicine industries.

Lavandula angustifolia, known as true lavender or English lavender, was until recently considered the hardiest and most fragrant species. It is a shrubby, semi-evergreen perennial with long narrow leaves, which explains its species name, *angustifolia,* meaning "narrow leaf." The common and genus names, lavender and *Lavandula,* were probably derived from the Latin word *lavare,* meaning "to wash." In Medieval Europe the washing women were known as lavenders.

Lavender may be the plant mentioned in the Bible as *spikenard* and the same plant that Mary used to anoint the feet of Jesus; *spike* may refer to its flower spikes. When stripped of flowers, the spike, or straw, has a variety of uses and contains the odor of lavender. *Nard,* another name for lavender, is Greek in origin. They gave it the name *Nardus* after the Syrian city of Naarda. There is also a species of lavender named spike lavender, *L. spica,* which is a broadleaved variety of the lavender shrub. Spike lavender grows in the mountainous areas of France and Spain and yields an essential oil known as spike oil.

English lavender, grown in farms throughout England, is arguably the most aromatic, possessing the greatest delicacy of scent and commanding the highest price. These farms were once extensive in England, but with the growth and expansion of London, coupled with the loss of land to food crops during World War I, the cultivation of lavender has diminished. Commercial growers now prefer a class of hybrids called the Intermediates, or Lavandins. A cross between *L. angustifolia* and *L. spica,* they produce the greatest yields of volatile oils, also known as essential oils, used in aromatherapy and cosmetics. Lavandin essential oil, however, is not as valuable as English lavender, and the seed is sterile.

The average English lavender is long-lived, having a flowering life of about ten years, with some plants living close to twenty years. Lavender grows best in dry, well-drained, sandy soil in full sun. It is considered a sustainable crop because it requires little or no fertilizer and pesticides. Although it is relatively disease and pest free, lavender is sensitive to root rot and requires good air circulation and excellent drainage. It likes to be cut back after blooming in order to promote compactness and vigor for the following season. In the cold winters of northern climates, lavender dies back completely.

To maintain crop purity, lavender is best propagated from softwood cuttings; plants grown from seed produce too much variability and are not true to type. While lavender is widely grown in gardens all over the world, garden escapees are found growing in the wild outside of its native habitat. Like most members of the mint family, lavender produces lots of volatile oils, which are responsible for the healing properties and distinctive scent when cut or crushed. The beauty, scent, and healing properties of lavender qualify it as the "queen of the herbs" for the herb garden. What cottage garden would be complete without her beauty and fragrance?

Rising on spikes above long, narrow leaves, lavender's violet blue flowers are borne in whorls. These are made up of five united petals and five united sepals. Their color epitomizes their name and is considered the standard for the color lavender. As an ornamental flower in the garden, it provides an extended season of colorful bloom. The flowers are best harvested at the height of summer. Dried flowers are used in floral arrangements, as an ingredient in potpourris and sachets, for ceremonial smudging, in smoking mixtures, and in candy or herbal tea.

Lavender is a feast for the olfactory senses. Although it has a long history of use in French cuisine, lavender has only recently found its way into American recipes. The traditional French seasoning known as *herbes de Provence* has been updated by American chefs, who added lavender to the classic blend of savory, fennel, basil, and thyme. Lavender brings a uniquely sweet flavor with balsamic undertones to many foods. It is also a spice that pairs well with goat and sheep milk cheeses, and it can be used as a dry rub for barbeque or as a substitute in most recipes that call for rosemary. The French are also known for their lavender syrup, an extract made from the flowers that adds a hint of floral character to baked goods. Each year lavender shows up more and more at farmer's markets and at lavender festivals throughout the United States, and it is becoming an important tourism attraction.

Cherished by beekeepers, lavender's abundant nectar yields a high-quality honey. The symbiotic relationship between lavender and honeybees is critical, as essential or volatile oil production increases with pollination. Pollinated flowers produce significantly more volatile oils.

Lavender flowers, cultivated extensively in France, Italy, and England, are primarily distilled for their essential oils. As the demand for lavender essential oil increases, countries like China and Australia are getting in on the action by boosting their production. One acre of *L. angustifolia* can produce up to 1,800 pounds of dried flowers, which results in about two gallons of essential oil. Oil yields can vary considerably from season to season, and the Hitchin family, which grows Lavender at Cadwell Farm in England, estimates that sixty pounds of fresh flowers yields sixteen fluid ounces of oil. The spirit or essence of lavender is expressed through its essential oil. As mentioned, it is used as a perfume, a medicine, and an ingredient in cosmetic preparations.

The historic use of lavender has been well documented for over two thousand years. The Egyptians, Phoenicians, and Arabians used it as a perfume and in the mummification process. When King Tutankhamun's tomb was opened in 1922 after being sealed for over three thousand years, traces of lavender could still be detected. (Lavender oil is still used in the embalming process, mostly in third-world countries, and this use is increasing.) It was used in Spain in landscaping, in Iran to treat burns, in England to scent linens and repel insects, and in Rome for scented baths. It is so effective as an antimicrobial that glove makers in sixteenth-century France, who were licensed to perfume their wares with lavender, didn't contract cholera. It is also an effective insect repellent. Seventeenth-century grave robbers, who washed in a formulation containing lavender known as "Thieves," rarely contracted the deadly plague that was caused by fleas.

Lavender essential oil is the one most widely used in aromatherapy, a healing technique that uses essential oils to relieve physical and psychological imbalances. It is one of the few essential oils that can be applied "neat," or undiluted, directly on the skin. The essential oil is steam distilled, using the whole plant when in flower. The result is a versatile oil with a pleasant aroma, used to make a wide variety of products, such as lotions, creams, body butters, massage oils, bath oils, bath salts, soaps, shampoos, deodorants, salves, balms, and air fresheners.

Because steam distillation is an expensive process that requires vast amounts of fresh plant matter, many small-scale producers use floral waters, or hydrosols, instead of pure essential oils. Hydrosols are by-products of the steam distillation process that produces essential oils. Less concentrated that essential oils, floral waters contain many of the same qualities but in a milder form.

The medicinal properties of lavender are many. Its herbal actions are antibacterial, antidepressant, antispasmodic, carminative, emmenagogue, hypotensive, nervine, and rubefacient. (Please see the section at the end of this book, titled "Herbal Actions," for a definition of these terms.) Lavender infusions (water-based extracts), essential oils, and hydrosols are used to treat burns, skin inflammations, minor abrasions, and insect bites.

It increases circulation to the skin and may help relieve rheumatic pain. Herbal tea made from lavender leaves and flowers relaxes and restores the nervous system to promote sleep and relieve tension, anxiety, and stress-related headaches, especially when the cause is overstimulation and nervous exhaustion. It is also beneficial in the treatment of digestive disorders and depression. The aroma of lavender is relaxing and uplifting, and it acts as a mild sedative for the central nervous system.

As mentioned previously, lavender is a member of the mint family, formerly called Labiatae, now known as Lamiaceae. The flowers of many mint family plants have two petals that form an upper and lower lip, and these were thought to resemble the female labium. This fold that surrounds women's genital organs comprises the labia majora and labia minora. The word *Labiatae* is derived from this anatomical term.

While women may be especially fond of lavender, the attractiveness of this plant is not limited to just women, however, for it is the receptive frequency of the feminine that attracts both men and women alike. While lavender may have been much sought after by Victorian royalty and grown in the garden of many a queen, the love of lavender is not limited to status, era, or region. The magic and power of this herb continue to unfold in our midst.

THE DIVINATION

At the edge of the meadow, in a clearing by the bay, lies a cottage where your ancestors once lived and played. It is empty now, but beckons to you, beneath the light of the full summer's moon. Behind this cottage is a garden, an ancient Medicine Wheel Garden. Lavender lines the path and will show you the way. And when you find yourself standing in the garden of your life, stop and ask, "What is the most appropriate medicine for me at this time?" Then prepare yourself to receive. For what you are really asking is to become more receptive. It is through receptivity, acceptance, and allowing that we are able to embrace both sides of our dualistic natures. The divine feminine *allows all things*. In the process of integrating our inner feminine and masculine, we learn how to navigate between unity and duality. While we long for unity, duality serves as one of our greatest teachers. Duality is a divine mirror.

The receptive qualities of the feminine are represented by the fluid quality of water and the emotions. Water is also an excellent conductor of sound. The feminine is constantly filling, overflowing, giving, and emptying, a cycle that allows endless receiving. Her energy is capable of dissolving all the obstacles that keep us separate from each other and from the whole. We can reach the guidance of the devas only when the devas can reach us, and the devas can reach us only when we are receptive. Receptivity is an open door where we forget ourselves completely and we are truly able to listen.

It is through the receptive feminine that our spirit descends into duality and we are born in the physical realm of human male and female form. Every thing, person, planet, animal, plant, and mineral is born of duality. It is in this spark created by the joining of opposites that new life is created. It is also through the receptive frequency of the feminine that we continue our journey from matter back to spirit, as matter simply changes form and spirit is eternal. The path from unity to duality and back again is the same, and we have made this journey many times, albeit not always consciously. Death and rebirth are two sides of the same mirror and do not always necessitate being born or dying in a physical body. In truth we are multidimensional beings traveling between dimensions while at the same time learning to navigate beyond even these realms of which we speak. Yoga teaches us that the wisdom of duality that exists in our physical form is expressed through the opposing structures of the body that create the foundation from which to open. Becoming more receptive and opening our hearts and minds will help us to receive the guidance we need to make the transition consciously.

Duality is like a smoking mirror. Your perception of the world creates the illusion. The smoking mirror teaches us not only to embrace our shadow, but also to accept light and shadow as two ends of the same spectrum. This is the mirror where we see the reflection of our self in others. We have all originated from the same source and are all unique expressions of that source. If you have become too invested in your ideas of what is right and what is wrong, then it is time to divest yourself of this illusion. The unified whole of your existence cannot be separated into the "good" and the "bad." The more you battle darkness, the more empowered it becomes. The more you deny it, the more empowered it becomes. What is not said carries just as much weight as what is. As the light grows lighter, the darkness grows darker. Look inside of yourself to accept all that you are. Only then can the world be transformed.

Inner peace is the experience of becoming neutral within duality. Neutrality is the unblocked flow of receptivity and emanation. This concept is perfectly represented in the symbol of the Tao. The yin polarity flows into the yang, and the yang into the yin. Duality provides the contrast by which we have an experience in physical form. Without the bitterness, could you distinguish the sweet? Duality is the expression of impermanence, and through acceptance we learn to ride the waves.

Perhaps the reason you are seeking the medicine of lavender is because you have become frustrated in your attempts to create positive change in the world, and the world is not responding with positive change. Perhaps you are proactive but have forgotten to take the time to be receptive to inner guidance. You are trying to create a world through your good works that will never exist. This doesn't mean that you should cease taking action for positive change; what it means is that if you would simply accept the darkness inside of yourself, then there would be no need for the darkness to be acted out in the world around you. Accept it for what it is, and there will be no more battles to be won. You are as capable of giving death as you are of giving life. When you repress this part of yourself and restrict others from acting by issuing laws that are not natural laws, you get a world in chaos.

Our world is presently in a state of chaos for this very reason. It is not a bad thing, only nature's attempt to keep the forces balanced and a tremendous opportunity for growth. If you don't like what is happening in your world, look inside. This is the place where change occurs. The Shift of the Ages has been initiated in this very place. It is through the doorway of your heart that you will shift into the next dimension, and fully into the fourth dimension of nonlinear time, and from there into yet other dimensions. This is already happening for many of you who have been working to clear the smoke of physical illusion. Many others are choosing not to make the shift at this time. You can only accept that this is their choice, for it is in the choosing that we find our empowerment, no matter what that looks like. There would be no free will without duality in which to choose one or the other. We are empowered through our choices, which is the foundation for the Law of Attraction. Each seeker will find his or her answer reflected in the divine mirror. The earth holds no judgment of our choices and will receive all that she has created back into her fold. She has chosen well.

The paradox of unity is that like and unlike are the same. Opposites are identical but different in degree. Only when we activate the dimensions of ourselves that have lain dormant will the degrees of paradox become reconciled. Everything that is manifest has two sides. We can see this exquisite manifestation in the pairs of opposites that reside all around us in nature. Poison ivy may cause us to itch and burn, but the remedy, jewelweed, grows right next to the ivy. Lavender may clean and soothe and fill our senses, but it demands a very specific environment in which to grow. Let us choose to throw our seeds into the fertile soil that has been prepared for us so we may be blessed with an abundant harvest.

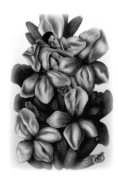

THE DEVA SPEAKS

I was conceived in the heavens and seeded on Earth. My herstory is contained within the female hormone of estrogen. I am "as above, so below." Sung into existence, I am the music of the spheres and descend on the spectrum of light known as the violet ray. While you are only just beginning to hear my song, you have perceived the complexity of my essence through your senses of taste and smell. Everything that can be perceived with one of the senses can also be perceived by all of the other senses. What can be smelled and tasted can also be heard. This principle applies to the song that exists within all of nature. My music contains the entire major and minor keys found within the circle of fifths. My harmonies are exquisite. The lips of my petals are formed in such a way to perfectly sing you this song. Every song ever sung on this beautiful Earth, beneath its heavenly stars, throughout all the ages and on every continent, has indeed been heard. These are the songs that have called me to be with you now so that we may be in service to each other.

Bathe in me, eat of me, breathe of me deeply. I give to you all of my medicines for your journey, but my greatest medicine of all is the knowledge that you were seeded by the stars and to the stars you will return. The legend of my song is written in the stars and lives in the constellation Cygnus, the Swan. The time is coming when your Earth will be held in the galactic center of the universe. At that time, you will experience a spontaneous combustion of beliefs. Listen carefully to that of which I speak. You must fully integrate the duality of this world before achieving the next, where there is no separation, only illumination. If you look closely at my flowers, you can perceive their separation. In a similar manner, you have overscrutinized your separation from All That Is. Understand that this separation lives only in your perception. Just as you are seeking union with the divine, I am also seeking union with you. We are destined to make the journey together across the Milky Road so that we may take our place among the stars.

Bend your ear close to my lips so that I may sing to you and you may hear the song of my essence. Learn to relax with the help of my medicine so that I may support you on the deepest level. As you relax you will become more receptive, and this will make your journey through the duality of this world so much easier. Quiet your mind so that I might speak to you sweetly of your magnificence.

You and I are separate from each other only by degrees of vibration, as are your worlds of spirit and matter. When you shift, I shift, and together we will transcend our current forms. As my separation from you lessens, my separation from the Central Sun, whose light I am becoming, also lessens. In this way we are lifting each other to the New Earth. You may look at me as a great teacher and say, "But we are many and you are only one." And I would reply that we are not separate, the many or the few, and the place where we come together in love knows neither hot nor cold, no night or day, only eternal love. For love is not absolute but on a spectrum of frequency, and this is the direction toward which you are moving.

The world around you is not necessarily moving as quickly in this direction, but you who have chosen love are accelerating toward this light. As you ascend you will discover more and more love. I emanate color to you through my love for you. I am on a spectrum of color; I heal you with my color because all the other colors are present in me. I operate on a sliding scale, and as you come into relationship with me, I bring you a little closer to the vibrational frequency of the pure essence of your soul. Would you laugh if I told you that you have a lavender soul? Transformation is simply transmuting one state of consciousness on the spectrum to another within the laws of duality. In other words, matter may be transformed only into other forms of matter, and thought into other forms of thought, and consciousness into other forms of consciousness. This is my medicine for you through my vibratory frequencies of light, sound, and color: your transformation. I wish not for you to change into a lavender flower or for you to become a deva in a light body as I am, for you have your own light body into which to evolve. It is my desire to assist you on your journey to become the body of light that contains an evolved human consciousness, for desire still lives in us both as a lavender flame.

Currently you are in a dense body of matter that contains a degree of darkness or shadow. This darkness is also within your consciousness. I hold open a door for you so that you may move more toward your light bodies by accepting the entire spectrum of who you are and who you are becoming. This is why you are hearing a lot about dimensional realities. You live in a dimensional reality and are transmuting your current reality into a new one, into a reality of love, into the reality of a New Earth.

You may ask me, "What is the nature of duality?" I would answer you that duality *is* nature. Even your scientists in their theories of the nature of light and matter have confirmed the dualistic nature of all of life. I operate on the violet frequency of light. It is on this frequency that you are able to view and contact the devas. Much insight has been gained in the reduction of matter to its smallest parts, but this way of thinking has also limited the view. You think of matter as made up of separate particles. It is actually a continuous field of light. When you look at an entire field of my vibrant, waving wands of color, the sensation you feel will connect you to the heart of this truth. Although my physical wands are waving as the result of an unseen force, and one seems solid and the other invisible, this dualism is an illusion. Step into the picture and feel the wind at your back. What is seen, or solid, is on one side of the mirror and what is unseen, or invisible, is on the other. Both are part of a unified field.

While duality is governed by opposite poles, with the positive pole vibrating at a higher frequency, the tendency of nature, of which you and I are a part, is to gravitate in the direction of the positive pole. By nature it is the dominant pole. You have many bodies: physical, mental, spiritual, and emotional. All of your bodies are influenced by the law of polarity, and all are moving in the positive direction of influence. I am this influence on your life simply because you have chosen to get to know me by picking up this book and reading this far into it. I am communicating my vibration to you by emanating the violet lavender ray.

This frequency contains within it both the masculine and feminine qualities of light that you have identified as blue and pink. Through your conscious and unconscious receptivity, you are receiving my positive influence. The more conscious and receptive you become to my frequency, the more your life unfolds in light and beauty. Stand in the cottage garden for just a moment, even if it is only in your powerful imagination, and behold my scent, my color, and my beauty: *for I am but a mirror.* When you choose to be in my presence and to use my medicine in any and all of the myriad forms in which it is available, you raise your vibration one degree at a time, until finally you will see that we stand together in the same field, warmed by a Central Sun. No longer a slave to your unconscious mind, you are waking to the truth of who you really are. In seeing this truth, you will lift all of humanity with the purity of who you are becoming, no different than I have been lifted and am now holding open the door for you, my beloveds.

Thought is one of the most powerful tools of transformation that you have. Know that your thoughts may be transmuted and transformed through the same law of polarity that applies to matter, and that you can raise all of your bodies—mental, spiritual, emotional, and physical—into the frequency of love. In the same manner the elementals from which you are made are being transmuted, along with the devic worlds, all of which exist on the same frequency spectrum. No longer of two minds, you will discover that the intelligence you have always thought of as being seated in the brain is actually an intelligence of the heart. It is through the inner chambers of this heart that you will be transformed.

Here is the key I wish to give you at this time. The moment of union when reconciliation between the pairs of opposites is achieved will be the same moment when you shift through the portal of your heart center into a fully conscious human being. The point of union where the pairs of opposites meet is the point that transcends duality. When you gaze into my tiny flowers made up of five united petals you will shift into the fifth dimension of consciousness, and the next four dimensions will be made available to you. The nine seeds of transformation for this shift into the nine dimensions have been sown. This shift in consciousness is being activated by my life-force energy on your planet at this very moment. The map to the garden lies in the spiral patterns that exist in all of physical creation, from the tiniest atom to the largest star system. The spiral *is* the path home to your multidimensional self. It can be seen in the whorl of my flowers, which mirrors the star clusters within your own spiral galaxy. You are not separate from All That Is. We are all star beings.

These nine seeds of transformation are rooted in the earth through my medicine, which feeds, nourishes, nurtures, and sustains you. You have only to receive it. When these seeds are warmed by the Central Sun and watered by the pure human emotion of love, they will begin to sprout and grow. And when new ground is breaking and new life raises its head above the fertile soil of your desire, you will find that you are standing on a New Earth.

Lavender Song

I've got to find me
some lavender honey
down where the mountains
roll sweetly to the sea

Breathe in deeply
perfumed lips are speaking
of a mystery beyond
what these eyes can see

In lavender hills
'neath a halo of stars
an ocean of longing
is calling from afar

And when she washes
over you sweetly
we will be dreaming
our new home by the sea

THEA SUMMER DEER

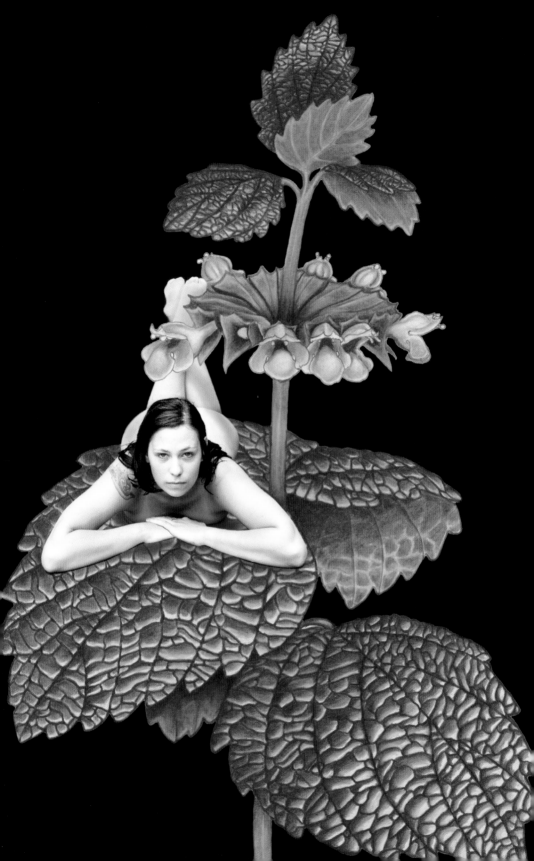

Lemon Balm

Melissa officinalis

Alignment

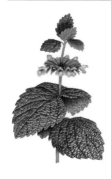

Melissa officinalis, more commonly known as lemon balm, has small flowers full of nectar in late summer, which honeybees find irresistible. *Melissa* is the Greek word for bee, which favors lemon balm above all other herbs. *Balm* is short for balsam, a word used to describe many aromatic plants. Lemon balm, a true summer essence, has a fragrant lemony odor when bruised and a distinctive lemony flavor. The species name, *officinalis,* indicates that lemon balm has a long history of use as a medicine. Paracelsus, a sixteenth-century physician and alchemist who desired immortality, called it the "elixir of life." Lemon balm is associated with both bees and balm, but it should not be confused with bee balm, *Monarda didyma.*

Lemon balm is a perennial herb in the Lamiaceae family of mints and native to the mountainous areas of southern Europe and the Mediterranean. It was introduced to the south of England around the tenth century, where it was known simply as balm, and it is now naturalized throughout northern Europe and parts of North America. Arabians may have been the first to introduce lemon balm to Europe. It was a valued part of the Arabian materia medica for hundreds of years and originally introduced to them by the Greeks, who valued it in trade. The plant can grow up to two feet in height, dies back in winter, and under ideal conditions is self-seeding. Melissa is an attractive plant with pale yellow flowers that turn pale lilac or white as they mature. The leaves are heart-shaped with serrated margins and a shiny, wrinkled texture.

Lemon balm is best grown in fertile, moist soil and mulched in the winter. It prefers cooler, partially shaded areas, but will grow in full sun, as long it doesn't become too hot at summer's peak. Easy to grow from seeds sown with a fine layer of soil covering them in the early spring or fall, it can also be started from stem cuttings and root divisions. Because it self-sows freely and spreads rapidly, it can quickly become invasive. An appropriate sign in a garden of lemon balm might be, "May all your weeds be wildflowers." It can also be easily grown indoors as a potted herb. Insects are not usually a problem with lemon balm due to the volatile oil contained in the leaves, which acts as a natural insect repellent. In fact, the freshly crushed leaves can be rubbed on the skin to help repel mosquitoes. Frequent trimming encourages branching and results in a fuller, bushier plant, and a handful of leaves can be harvested for fresh use once or twice a week. When larger amounts are desired for drying, it is best to harvest twice during the season, as the plant comes into bloom.

Lemon balm is a culinary, cosmetic, and medicinal herb, and is highly prized for its sweet-smelling oil. During the seventeenth century, Carmelite nuns produced their famous Carmelite water, also known as *eau de mélisse des Carmes-boyer,* an extract made from lemon balm and other herbs. It was used to aid digestion, increase mental clarity, and treat nervous disorders. The exact proportions of the original recipe remain a mystery.

While lemon balm is a lovely addition to potpourris, this minty-lemony herb can also add a dash of honeyed sweetness and vibrant flavor to a wide range of culinary dishes. Used in place of lemon peel, it can be made into a marinade or lemon balm pesto, added to salad dressing, and used to flavor a host of desserts including cookies, cakes, fruit dishes, jellies, syrups, and poppy seed bread. Lemon balm makes a refreshing herbal tea, both hot and iced, and it is an ingredient in Chartreuse and Bénédictine liqueurs and in the fortified wine vermouth. Many chefs prefer to use vermouth, dry or sweet, as a cooking wine because of its stability and extended shelf life. Lemon balm can be used in a *bouquet garni* (herb bundle) for soups, stews, and sauces. Fresh sprigs make a decorative, fragrant garnish.

As a medicinal herb, lemon balm has mild sedative properties. It is an effective sleep aid and may relieve depression. It is carminative and a tonic for stress-related digestive problems. Steeped in wine, it was used in ancient Greece and Rome, and in Europe in the late 1600s, for nervousness, memory impairment, and depression. In addition to its sedative and carminative properties, lemon balm's primary actions are diaphoretic and febrifuge. Fresh leaves or the diluted essential oil added to a bath can act as an emmenagogue and alleviate painful or delayed menses, probably due to its rosmarinic acid content. For this reason it should be avoided during pregnancy. A hot tea made from dried or fresh leaves is a trusted folk remedy that causes sweating, reduces fevers, and relieves gas and bloating. As a mild vasodilator it can reduce heart rate and lower blood pressure. According to the London Dispensary of 1696, it had a reputation for promoting longevity. It has been documented that a number of people who drank an infusion of the fresh leaf tea daily lived to be over a hundred.

The popularity of lemon balm during Shakespeare's lifetime (1564–1616) is evident in his plays, where it is used to anoint and consecrate kings, as well as to alleviate a king's suffering from sorrow and grief. Nicholas Culpepper, a seventeenth-century astrologer and herbalist, classified lemon balm as a nurturing herb that belonged to the sign of Cancer. He also observed that it could be used to dry damp conditions of the lungs and stomach.

Lemon balm is widely used in aromatherapy and referred to as melissa by aromatherapists. It is one of the most expensive essential oils because it takes approximately three tons of plant material to yield one pound of the essential oil. Even though it is costly, melissa is one of the most valuable aromatherapy oils because it directly affects the autonomic nervous system to alleviate depression. The volatile oil contains monoterpene, citral, and other constituents that have been shown to possess strong antibacterial and antiviral qualities. Added to carrier oil for use in massage therapy, it is very effective for calming the nerves, promoting rest, and lifting the spirits. Melissa is used to treat attention deficit disorder, as it is also calming to the nervous system and reduces irritability and excitability.

The International Fragrance Association (IFRA) greatly affected the use of melissa oil in perfumery when the organization banned its use in 2006 as a result of studies that classified it as a weak sensitizer, meaning it could cause skin irritation in some individuals. In 2008 the IFRA amended the ban to a concentration restriction. For those working in the aroma trade, the studies were seen as faulted and the regulations nonsensical, imposed by unelected officials who had little in-depth working knowledge or experience with melissa oil. Safety-oriented organizations that take choices away from consumers foster a dependency on experts to tell us what is safe, rather than conducting sound research and making it available to the general public.

Melissa is a popular girl's name and is also the name of a Greek nymph who was the protector of bees and taught the uses of honey to the Greek gods and goddesses. Bees became the symbol of the nymphs, and one story tells of how the nymph Melissa cared for the infant Zeus while he was being hidden from his father. She fed him honey to keep him alive until her protector role was discovered and she was turned into a lowly insect. Zeus later took pity on her and turned her into a honeybee so that she would forever be involved in the making of honey. In Greek mythology, the nymphs were seen as neither good nor evil, but as providers of skills and training and as the teachers of civilizing behaviors. They were dangerous when provoked but possessed the dignity of a goddess.

Thousands of years ago in ancient Ephesus, in what is known today as Turkey, the bee symbolized the Great Goddess. The mother goddesses Rhea, Cybele, Demeter, and Artemis who served the Great Goddess were in turn served by priestesses who had the title of Melissa. Artemis, who appeared in Ephesus, was not a virgin as she was later depicted in Greece. The term "virgin" in Jungian psychology has its roots in an older mythology, and a virgin goddess, in this more classical sense, means "complete unto oneself," or sovereign, whether she has had sex or not.

Lemon balm was sacred in the temples and used by beekeepers to keep their honeybees supplied with nectar. The honeybee was believed to be the form a human soul took upon dying and returning home to the hive, or sacred source. Honey was important to the Minoan culture in Crete, where the bee signified the life that comes from death, a symbol similar to that of the scarab for the Egyptians. Both cultures used honey for embalming the dead and oriented their temple sites to the rising of the great star Sirius. Sirius was the star of the goddess Innana in Sumeria, and its rising ended a month-long ritual, during which honey was gathered and fermented into mead, which was then drank to celebrate Innana's return from the underworld and the beginning of a new year.

THE DIVINATION

If you are longing for respite from the frantic and hurried pace, then quickly enter the Medicine Wheel Garden and look for sweet Melissa's calming face. When you find her there, crush the scented leaves gently between your fingers and breathe the purity of her essence. She reminds us that we can choose to live life with purity and simplicity. She heals the wound in our collective human psyche from the will to survive and the drive to succeed. We can no longer separate spirit and body on this journey to the light. We must bring all of ourselves into the center of the Medicine Wheel Garden.

All of the ways that we have explored our powers of creation and have manipulated our universe, from artificial light to microwave technology and the creation of ever more harmful chemicals, are not in alignment with the rhythms of nature. The disconnection from nature that we experience when we live in artificial environments is causing the spirit to flee the body. This isolation is one of the major causes of depression, and the statistics are staggering. While it has been necessary to explore the split into duality in our journey of self-discovery, it is now time to align within a more expanded dimension of reality. Our survival gene, which had not been fully hooked up, is now waking up, as more strands of DNA are "turning on" so that we can know what it is to live beyond survival. No one knows where this new hookup will take us or what it will look like. Lemon balm can help to calm and center us as we align with the new energies unfolding on our planet.

Alignment is one of the keys of manifestation. It is an energetic configuration that frees us of limiting beliefs and opens the doors of possibility into the bigger room of ease and abundance. The room of limitation was a place from which to open the door, and the key is made of interconnectedness. Judgment and fear will fall away once we turn the key, and past limitations will no longer be viewed as good or bad. Our ability to manifest ease and abundance and the quality of our experience are directly related to our connection with nature. Nature provides for all of our needs, and when we are in alignment, nothing is excluded. Alignment is where we get hooked up, keyed in, downloaded. Lemon balm supports us in aligning our desires with our passion for the truth. We can make our needs our wants, and our wants our needs. This alchemical key of manifestation transforms insatiable greed and desire for excess into the divine nectar of fulfillment, where nothing is ever wasted and we always have enough. When we learn how to receive instead of take and how to give back as much as we have received, then we enter into the divine presence and the larger room of ease and abundance. There is no limit to what we can create when we are in alignment with the divine presence.

Learning how to align oneself requires daily practice. The form of this practice could look like anything that we show up for consistently while holding the intention of aligning with a higher vibratory pattern. It could be simply sitting with a straight spine and paying attention to the breath moving in and out of our body, an artistic expression of some kind, a daily walk in the garden or gardening itself, a more disciplined form of meditation, or rigorous athletic training. Regardless, it will be an ever-constant and changing dance, as sure as nature changes with the seasons and the cycles of gestation, birth, growth, maturity, decline, and death. The flexibility to have a practice that also grows and changes builds a kind of resilient inner strength that helps us to bend with the winds of change in our lives.

Drinking a cup of fresh lemon balm tea daily when it is in season would be a wise practice for fostering longevity. Adding healthy years to one's life could be one way of practicing alignment. When we align with the laws of nature, the secrets of the universe are revealed. It is as simple as taking the first step of entering the Medicine Wheel Garden, where we meet and align with our plant spirit allies. As we work creatively with nature, we will discover that the doorway into the next dimension is through nature itself. We could not and would not exist in this dimension without the forms of nature that have evolved concurrently and in harmonic resonance with our expression of humanity. Nature has been at this for a very long time. Human intelligence will take a quantum leap when we become fully conscious of this partnership and aligned with plant intelligence.

When you begin to partner with lemon balm, you may feel a strange attraction to this medicine plant. Allow its calming influence to recalibrate and align your feeling center with your nervous system. The attraction you are feeling is similar to the attraction that bees have for this plant. When you first hear the sound of bees in the garden or feel them on your skin, if you are not familiar or have not established a relationship with them, you may feel fear. Fear is one of the first human emotions and lives in the lower charkas. It has informed your survival. As you allow yourself to journey with the spirit of lemon balm, she will help you to release all preconceived notions and will lead you to the sweet reward of nectar. Bees have a certain level of organization and communication that allows them to produce nectar for the gods and goddesses. The bees are in alignment with their sacred purpose. Be the god or goddess whom their nectar feeds, and know the truth of your own divinity.

The importance of lemon balm in our evolution and its role in the health of the bees, the Melissas, that love it cannot be underestimated. Most of lemon balm's magical powers can be attributed to its association with the insect Melissas. The health of the bees is at risk, and we would do well to pay close attention to their decline. Beekeepers of old rubbed lemon balm on the inside of their hives to keep the bees from swarming and leaving the hive. They also planted lemon balm all around the hives to encourage the honeybees to return. They understood the benefit of a healthy partnership.

We are returning in a similar manner to the hive of our sacred purpose, calling in the spirits of the sacred plants to aid us in our transformation. If we calm and focus our minds with the aid of lemon balm and align ourselves with the visible and invisible forces of nature, we will discover that what flows within us is the taste of something very sweet, a nectar that pours from the source, the divine elixir of a fully embodied human experience. What previously existed in the realm of mythological gods and goddesses is now unfolding in our midst.

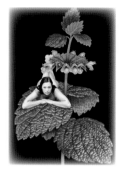

THE DEVA SPEAKS

What will you align yourselves with, my beloveds—the truth of the wholeness and interconnectedness of all of life? From the farthest star to the light at the core of the atoms from which you are made, from the void of deep space to the darkness of the grave, what degree of separation would you prescribe for that which is inseparable? A multitude of galaxies exists within your body and mirrors the stars in the heaven of your Earth. I am an energetic plant and hold open the door to the energetic portals within you. You have named these portals *chakras,* and by aligning yourselves within this system you will be able to walk into yet other dimensions and learn to align with even greater systems.

The tiniest insect is no less than you are, and this is the truth of carbon-based life on your planet. These ones who crawl the closest to the earth have great messages for you. When you hear the buzzing of the sacred ones called Melissas, they are tuning the vibrational frequencies of Earth to support the life that I call forth. When you hear the cicadas and the tree frogs, they are making music more profound than any human symphony has ever produced. Your hearing is limited to a certain bandwidth and frequency of sound, but theirs is tuned to the music of the spheres. Even your sound-capturing devices are not sophisticated enough to record their music. Their music calls the rain and the thunder. It directs the wind. It wakes up the mycelium that creates a network larger and more sophisticated than any Internet system devised by humans. Your technology, microwaves, and other forms of radiation that you are unleashing on the planet are giving death to these sensitive ones. From this you are learning how you are both creator and destroyer. You are learning just how powerful you really are. This knowledge will be available to you when you align yourselves with the subtle frequencies of nature, which you have been too busy to notice.

"How can we do this?" you would ask of me. And I will answer: *Be wholly human. Embrace the whole of life that includes death. Live and die in alignment with the natural laws, and know the creative power of your thoughts and visions.*

You have sought to survive because you believed it was the antidote to death. But death has not escaped you. Death, as you know it, does not exist for me. What you perceive as death is only a transfiguration of living matter into spirit. My roots are perennial, as are yours. Through our roots we transmute death and decay into light and living matter. One does not exist without the other. You are healing your ancestors, as am I healing you. First there was darkness, and then there was light, and to darkness you shall return. In this moment of divine presence, you are in a cycle of light. Journey well into this light, for this is a profound moment of in-lightenment. When you are fully aligned within the laws of nature, when spirit is infused in body, you will travel seamlessly between the worlds of life and death, bringing the light of spirit back into the darkness of matter, and you will choose the creation of your next vehicle. Matter is mother, and mother is Earth, and Earth is your physical body animated by breath. This is what is meant by a New Earth—your body made new when it becomes fully infused with spirit. When you are aligned with the laws of nature, the spirit in all matter will be readily apparent, and these spirits, of which I am one, are ecstatic that you have joined the dance and are ready to step into the light.

Bring yourselves into alignment with your Earth through the elements of earth, fire, water, and air. I contain all of the elements, and when you eat and drink of my body, I will bring you into alignment with your sacred purpose as a human being. There is more yet to discover, more to awaken within your codes. Many have fallen asleep and will fall back into the earth from which they have come. Nothing is ever wasted. All that your heart desires awaits your alignment with the light and the energy that I transmit to you through my own body of light. I am singing to you with the top notes of my sacred scent of the promise of nectar. Drink deeply, for this is my gift.

Some of you do not know what your gifts are, and for some your gifts have been perverted due to misalignment. This is the source of your depressed energy. Receive my essence through your senses and learn how to create a dialogue with your Highest Self. When you become aware of the creative power of your thoughts and prayers and surrender your defenses, you will be guided and shown the gift that you carry—the gift that you are. I am asking you to see what an incredible gift you are to creation. When you self-realize through the integration of your Higher Self and reclaim what has been severed, all action taken from this new place of wholeness will be in the greater service of all creation.

Align yourself with what it means to be a fully present human, for you are standing at the galactic center of your universe. All the information contained in all the past ages is being made available to you at this time. During the acceleration toward the galactic center, many things have crumbled and fallen away. At the same time that your star system is quickening, you must learn to slow down. This is one of the paradoxes through which you are pulled back to the goddess. Calming the mind is of the utmost importance for aligning with the guidance system of your soul. My medicine will help you to align your nervous system with your spiritual purpose. In order to access all the memory in your genetic codes, you must enter into a receptive state. Some of these codes are very, very old, from a time when humanity moved at a much slower pace. As the light of your sun grows brighter and flares to impulse you, you will find yourself journeying deeper into the still darkness of the void from which all of creation has taken its birth. You are aligning with the totality of yourself as a human being, a multidimensional human being. Awaken! I am calling you back to the light. Align! All is in divine order. Activate! Become your Highest Self.

Melissa's Chant

I do among the gardens fly
Aligned with spirit as I die
Rising from the Goddess robes
To touch the hem of her abode
Aligned with spirit whole and healed
Grace and compassion now revealed
I fed the King and Queen of old
I tell a story yet to unfold
Of human form becoming light
Awakened from the longest night

And blessed with knowledge deep and vast
I gathered nectar from the past
To wake the strands of DNA
For the promise of a bright new day

THEA SUMMER DEER

Eau de Melissa

1¼ cups vodka
¾-inch piece angelica stem
3 tablespoons fresh lemon balm leaves
1 cinnamon stick
5 whole cloves
1 teaspoon nutmeg
1 tablespoon coriander seeds, crushed
1 tablespoon chopped lemon peel

Place all ingredients in a jar and cover with vodka. Make sure the jar is the right size so there isn't much room left at the top. Cap tightly. Let sit in a warm place, shaking daily, for approximately two weeks, preferably from new moon to full moon. Strain into a sterilized bottle and let stand for two weeks. Store in a cool, dark place and use within six months. Good for calming the nerves, lifting the spirits, and relieving bodily chills. Take one teaspoon as needed or add twenty to forty drops to a warm cup of lemon balm tea.

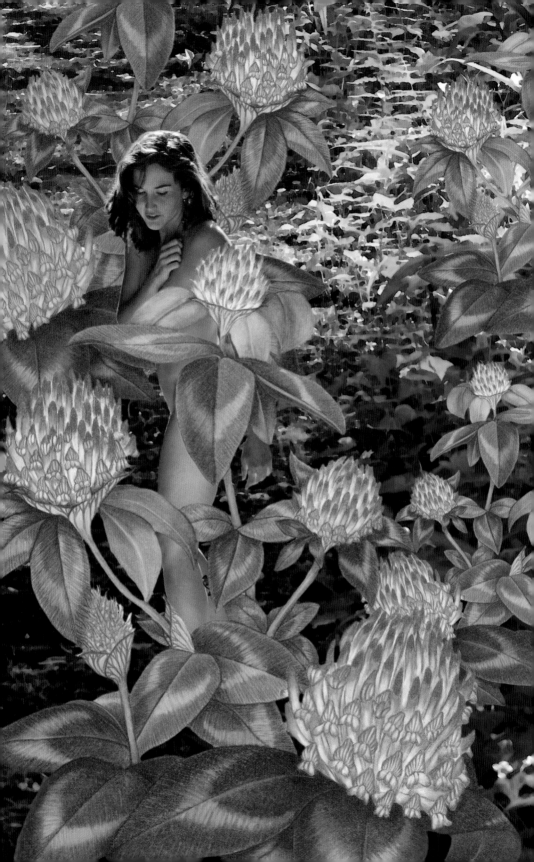

Red Clover

Trifolium pratense

Divine Nourishment

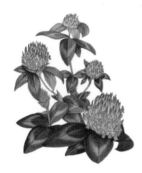

Red clover, *Trifolium pratense,* with its distinctive trefoil leaf, is one of several plants believed to be the original Irish shamrock. The shamrock is a symbol for Ireland and associated with the Christian symbol of the Holy Trinity. The species name, *Trifolium,* means "three leaves." As the Celtic symbol of perpetuity, the three leaves of the trefoil represent past, present, and future. In Gothic architecture the three-lobed or trifoliate pattern represent the Trinity. Red clover leaves may have also been the inspiration for the suit of clubs in playing cards.

Trifolium is a genus of about 250 recognized species in the Fabaceae, or pea, family. Its species name, *pratense,* describes its preferred habitat: meadows. An abundant dweller of fields, pastures, and meadows throughout temperate regions, red clover is native to Europe, central Asia, and northern Africa. Like most legumes, red clover is important ecologically as a nitrogen fixer. It has a symbiotic relationship with bacteria that colonize its root nodules, extracting nitrogen from the air and bringing it down to the earth, where it fixes in the soil. When tilled under, it continues to make nitrogen available to other plants in the garden. It is an excellent cover and rotation crop, as well as a valued green manure.

As concerns about water conservation and pollution from chemical fertilizers, herbicides, and lawn mower emissions increase, red clover is seeing more use as a grass alternative in lawns. It tolerates a wide range of growing conditions, requires little water or maintenance, and has deep roots that aerate the soil. Another excellent reason to plant red clover is that it has beautiful flowers that attract honeybees, butterflies, and other beneficial insects. It has a special relationship with the moth caterpillar *Coleophora deauratella,* which feeds on red clover exclusively and then encloses itself in a cocoon that closely resembles one of its tiny petals.

The name *red clover* is somewhat misleading. The flower head, which is approximately one inch across, is actually a cluster of tiny pink to purple pink florets. These florets are lighter toward the base of the flower head; they are never red. A short-lived perennial that prefers full sun, red clover blooms from late spring to midsummer. Both flowers and leaflets have a distinctively sweet, honeylike fragrance and flavor. The trifoliate leaves are made up of three hairy, ovate leaflets, two inches long, each with a distinct chevron-shaped mark pointing toward the tip. Leaves grow alternately along the stems, which are covered in fine hair, occasionally branched, and terminate in the flower head. The first leaves below the flower are sessile, or attached directly to the stem, along with several bracts, or modified leaves. The sessile leaflets of red clover are unusual among most clovers, and it is said that Saint Patrick taught that they symbolized the common "stalk" that unites all people.

After blooming, each flower forms a small seedpod with one or two heart-shaped seeds. The root system consists of a deep taproot and lateral roots radiating out from the crown. The lateral roots can be broken or divided to propagate new plants. Red clover is one of the world's oldest agricultural crops and is still extensively cultivated as animal fodder. Other common names arose as a result of this use: cow grass and cow clover. Research indicates that cattle or sheep that graze heavily on red clover can develop infertility issues due to its high phytoestrogen content. Wild red clover has always been an important food source for wild animals; game birds, small mammals, and browsers such as deer, elk, and moose eat both the seed heads and foliage.

Red clover provides wild and domestic animals with protein and has more microminerals than the other clover grasses. Red clover sprouts are rich in enzymes and contain a fair amount of nutritious, health-promoting vitamins, minerals, trace minerals, and chlorophyll. Red clover also has the distinction of being the official state flower of Vermont. Even though it is not a native of Vermont, but a European import, it is symbolic of Vermont's scenic countryside and its dairy farms in particular.

Not only cows appreciate the sweet taste of clover; Shakespeare mentions the "honey stalks" of red clover in *Titus Andronicus*.[1] Red clover petals are eaten raw in salads, and the flower head and aerial parts are dried, infused in hot water, and drank as a tea. The dried flower heads and seedpods can also be ground to make nutritious flour and combined with other ingredients. Red clover is considered a valuable survival food. Sprouted clover is an excellent way to get the nutritional benefits from this plant. A popular alternative to alfalfa sprouts, which they resemble, red clover sprouts have a sweet, mildly nutty flavor and last longer under refrigeration.

The recent trend toward gourmet microgreens has created a new market for this herb. Red clover microgreens have higher concentrations of nutrients than the mature plants. Smaller and more tender than baby lettuces, microgreens are more flavorful than sprouts and can be juiced or used to enhance salads, main dishes, and soups. In the fast-growing business of "functional foods," foods grown to increase disease-preventing properties or enhance health benefits beyond basic nutrition, microgreens like red clover look promising.

Isoflavones, one of the main chemical constituents of red clover, have been shown to interfere with estrogen receptors in humans. A particular type of isoflavone, genistein, is believed to be responsible for preventing some forms of cancer. Red clover is also one of the ingredients in Essiac tea, a North American Indian tea used to treat cancer.

It is important to remember that positive health benefits from ingesting plants are generally due to a subtle combination of phytochemicals. Ingesting isolated phytochemicals as opposed to the whole plant increases the likelihood of adverse reactions. Estrogen-like compounds can mimic the effect of endogenous estrogen (estrogen produced in the body) and act to either block estrogen receptor sites or boost estrogen in the system. The confusion and debate over whether or not to ingest phytoestrogens seems to stem from animal and in vitro research on isolated and concentrated isoflavones, but the relevance of this research to humans is not known. One theory is that in premenopausal women with high hormone levels, phytoestrogens block the estrogen receptor sites, which protects against certain cancers. After menopause, when estrogen levels are lower, phytoestrogens can act like estrogens, relieving menopausal symptoms. Phytoestrogens may also protect tissues from the cancer-causing effects of xenoestrogens, or estrogens found in commercially raised meat, dairy products, and environmental pollutants.

Traditionally, red clover has been used to help restore hormonal balance in women. It contains calcium and magnesium, which can relax the nervous system and improve fertility in women who are not ovulating due to high stress levels. It also has a balancing effect on the acid-alkaline level of the vagina. Red clover can potentially relieve symptoms of PMS and menopause, as well as alleviate problems associated with fibrocystic disease. It is best used as an infused tea made with the dried or fresh flowering tops.

An important medicinal herb, red clover's actions are alterative, expectorant, and antispasmodic. Alteratives restore the body and support a healthy metabolism by increasing nutrient absorption and the elimination of toxins. This action is not fully understood, and some people think of red clover as a blood cleanser. What it actually does is aid in the elimination of waste through the skin. It is a nourishing plant with an affinity for the skin and nervous system, and it has been used to treat chronic skin conditions such as psoriasis and childhood eczema. Red clover's combined expectorant and antispasmodic action makes it especially useful in the treatment of persistent spasmodic coughs and bronchitis.

The story of red clover would not be complete without acknowledging its dependency on bees. To produce seed, red clover must be cross-pollinated, and while it is most efficiently pollinated by bumblebees, it is a major nectar source for honeybees. To gather the nectar secreted at the base of the flower, the honeybee trips the petal doors by exerting pressure with its head. The amount of nectar secreted by the plant is determined by the available soil nutrients. Healthy soil means healthy plants and plenty of nectar for the bees.

Beekeepers who locate their hives in areas rich with clover can produce up to five hundred pounds of honey per acre in a good year. Farmers often contract with beekeepers to move their hives near pastures planted in clover in order to benefit from the increased seed production that occurs with increased bee activity. Bumblebee populations are diminishing due to a number of environmental factors, including the continued use of insecticides and a general decline in commercial beekeeping. This has led to a significant reduction of acreage in red clover seed production. Although red clover is vulnerable to bacterial, viral, fungal, and parasitic infestations, pollinator decline may also be a contributing factor to the condition known as "clover sickness." Without the honeybee there would be no clover honey, the most widely produced honey in the United States, Canada, Australia, and New Zealand.

Red clover honey is a magical elixir that is the result of the combined contributions of flowers, bees, and biochemistry. Honey made exclusively from red clover has a pale amber color and a subtle flavor. The medicinal value of red clover extends to the honey that it produces when used in its raw, unprocessed state. Far from being an empty sugar, red clover honey, like all raw honey, contains high levels of vitamins and minerals. The therapeutic properties of honey have been well documented throughout our human history and put to use by practically every culture and healing tradition in the world. These uses are not limited to physical ailments but are infused with spiritual meaning and written about in numerous scriptures and religious texts. The honey made from red clover holds the secret of divine nourishment.

THE DIVINATION

When you find yourself standing in a field of red clover at the center of the Medicine Wheel Garden, you have discovered the source of divine nourishment. This nourishment is not something necessarily obtained from food or by using the physical form of a plant; it comes from surrounding yourself with beauty, giving yourself in service, and receiving the nurturing of those who love you. It is nourishment on all levels of your being. These fields of clover that call to you are the fields of your childhood dreams, where you were cared for and nourished and had no thought of personal survival. When you find yourself in this field of red clover, take a moment to stop, see, and listen to something very magical taking place. It is the song of the bumblebee, and somewhere between the perfume and the music, you might find yourself moving to a new tune—drumming and dancing like a bee does with its wings to communicate the location and richness of a newly discovered source of nectar. It is the nectar of divine nourishment.

The expression "to be in clover" means to live a life of ease, abundance, and prosperity. It meant that after the fields were planted "in the clover" following the harvest, the hard work of the season was over. This is the new dance, the new song in our midst. It speaks of a worry-free life filled with the comfort of knowing that everything we need has already been richly provided for. The hard work is over, and the harvest is in. All the answers to all the questions about our continued existence and the right way to live on the earth have been right inside us all along. It only requires a shift in perspective to see the abundance of free energy that is available to us at this time. And for the first time in our human story, we are collectively beginning to hear this song and know the answers at a level that is tipping the scale toward mass enlightenment.

The truth is very simple. We are all interconnected, and there is no separating ourselves from that which conceives, births, and sustains us. It is not complicated or confusing, but we do get to choose, and that choice will determine the quality of our experience. The bee goddess, who loves her clover, is humming this very tune, this very truth. We are not separate from the elements that build and birth our material world. We have only to open our hearts and listen, open our mouths and sing, open our minds and receive this ancient wisdom. In this, we find harmony like bees working together in the hive, with a unified mind and a sense of purpose.

Red clover's gifts will balance and restore us to the original instructions with a few important new downloads. Hers is the wisdom of nourishment and grounding that allows us to know our spiritual work while residing in a physical body. When we are divinely nourished, we become the sacred beings that we were given life to be.

The chevron symbol that red clover so prominently displays is an esoteric symbol largely forgotten in its modern use on logos and as a military insignia.

It is an ancient symbol displayed on tombs in Egypt and above the tomb of Jesus. It is symbolic of the doorway to our heart center. This sacred geometric symbol was worn or displayed as a sign of protection for those who had accomplished a faithful work of service, which is exactly what the bees are doing as they gather honey in service to their queen. The chevron also represents the union of masculine and feminine. When the "V" is pointing down, two lines create the shape of the female opening, with the point being the male projection. It is the map the bees follow to enter red clover and receive her nectar.

Be curious about sex. Sexual curiosity is healthy and desirable. It is what guides you to the center of your being as the electrical circuit is completed between polarities. It is from this center that you will fly out and discover new nectar sources in the abundant fields of red clover that lie beyond the edge of space and time. The key is to learn how to become weightless and to fly. It is similar to the experience of orgasm, when you don't know what is beyond the door that is opening, but you go there anyway. It is a weightless place where for a moment the ego is suspended and nectar flows, giving up its scent through your body in the same way that a flower attracts its pollinator.

Be curious about the world of nature, for everything you eat and breathe is sex. Creation itself would not exist were it not for the masculine and feminine principles at work. The very wheel of life is based on these principles in their various forms. The sky above us: warming, raining, blowing, shining. The earth below us: solid, holding, supportive, nurturing. We are magical beings made up of the same thing as the earth and stars. The feminine principle of nurturing and nourishing is what gives birth to new seeds and new ideas, pollinated by the souls of those who have gone before and of those yet to come.

Divine nourishment is the domain of the Goddess. How lucky we are to be sitting in her lap. Who hasn't spent hours hunting in the grass for a four-leaf clover? But the truth is that every leaf of clover, every breath of life, brings us the good fortune of a charmed and prosperous life.

The number three represented by the trifoliate leaves is a powerful number. It appears in many different forms of symbolism and is significant to many of the world's religions. Long before it symbolized the Christian

Holy Trinity, the number three represented life, death, and rebirth. The Hindu Trinity of Brahman, Vishnu, and Shiva represents creator, preserver, and destroyer. Shiva, a major Hindu deity, is the destroyer and transformer who captivates, consolidates, and destroys. He is often depicted with the trident, an emblem of sovereignty. The trinity represents the divine in its threefold nature and function, with each aspect containing and including the others.

One of the most complex figures in Celtic mythology, the great sovereign queen, Morrigan, who was also the Triple Goddess of ancient Ireland, was seen as representing the three phases of a woman's life: maiden, mother, and crone. She gives life; she gives death; and she nurtures, nourishes, and devours. There are three vertical pillars in the Kabbalistic Tree of Life. The power of three can also be seen in the concept of chakras. The most well-known system in the East describes seven chakras. The configuration can be viewed as three above and three below, with each group forming a three-sided pyramid that together frame the heart at the core. This heart is a doorway, a stargate that is mirrored in the pyramids of Egypt, through which we can access other dimensional realities of creation. When two triangles are laid on top of each other in opposite directions, they create a hexagram.

The symbolism of the hexagram is extensive and includes the Merkabah and the balance between masculine and feminine, between heaven and earth, represented by two intersecting equilateral triangles that create a hexagon at the intersection. The cells of a beehive honeycomb are made up of hexagons, because this makes the best use of space and matter. Additional symbolism can be seen in the nine worlds of Norse mythology, in which chevrons composed the sides of a three-dimensional cube that was drawn in two dimensions.

The upper cube was blue and represented heaven; the lower cube was red and represented the underworld. Between the two was the three-dimensional reality of Middle Earth. Red clover is feeding us in this Middle Earth with her divine nourishment. Her roots know the underworld, and her crown knows the humming song that opens the heavens. When we have fully consumed the beauty of this world and have been divinely nourished by the medicine of red clover, we will have followed her map to the source—the source of nectar and of an abundant and prosperous life as we enter the New Earth.

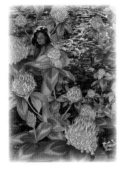

THE DEVA SPEAKS

Nourishment and assimilation of that nourishment on all levels is my prayer for you. My roots are nourished in the underworld, where darkness resides and life is transformed through death, decay, and rebirth. Although I am rooted in darkness and abundant among you, this darkness, death, and decay nourishes me, sustaining my production of an infinity of flowers, which hold pure nectar and beckon the vibrational frequency of the winged ones. This frequency awakens codes within you, codes of a new human who desires a New Earth. These souls among you in the buzzing form of bees come from the center of a hive constructed in sacred geometry. They are not of this world, but are here to serve our evolution, for without them neither you nor I would exist in our present forms. The subtle body they awaken in you is accessed through thought and feeling and is a measurable electromagnetic field. When you are divinely nourished, your electromagnetic fields resonate in harmony and match the vibration that your soul desires to create. Through thought and feeling you are creating your life, and in fact you are creating whole new worlds as you come into harmonic resonance with your soul.

Take time for yourself, for it takes time to truly nourish oneself. Take a moment to see and hear the magic that is taking place in the garden of your life. Magic buzzes all around you. Drink of its nectar and be completely fulfilled. The bee sings of a world where you have everything you need, and it sings of your divinity. For a moment, imagine that you pluck a sprig of red clover from the ground, hold its flower to your lips, and sip its divine nectar. Allow yourself to smell and taste the sweetness of this magic as you remember the sweetness of life.

When the bee comes to partake of me, this is my ecstasy. I have lived for this moment. Hold this thought for yourselves: *something is coming to sip from the flower of your divine essence.* It is a feeling unlike any you have ever known. Open yourselves to receive this feeling, for when it comes, it will be the moment in which your purpose as a human being throughout all your lifetimes is fulfilled. It will be the moment in which all karmic patterns dissolve and you are complete unto yourselves. That moment is now. Be nourished and nurture.

The world of magic is full of symbols. In the past, those meanings were revealed only to those who had been initiated. At this time in your human evolution, the mysteries are being unveiled to all who wish to receive them. Should you choose, you can now see what was previously unseen. This new perception comes from having received a new heart through many lifetimes of dismantling and reconstruction. The veils are growing thin due to the increasing light from both the solar and the Central Sun. The symbols of sacred geometry are reawakening your slumbering past and informing you from the future. By being conscious of and focusing on any one of these geometric symbols, you will be afforded the opportunity of initiation into its higher meaning. There is no more waiting for the knowledge of the ages to be revealed. One need only be willing to stop and see.

Interpretations of the divinity of the number three, or what you call the trinity, are dissolving as you leave the age of reason. Those who sought power through these interpretations and sought to keep hidden the truths of your divine origins are evolving souls no different from the rest. All interpretations have served your spiritual development. The hidden secrets of the Goddess contain many of the mysteries that have been kept from you. The masculine mysteries have also long suffered in their disconnection from the sacred source. Both of your polarities are longing for sacred marriage. When this marriage of God and Goddess takes place, a sacred third will be created. This birth will happen the moment that Old Earth separates from New Earth and the umbilical cord is cut.

How many times have you remade yourself in this one lifetime alone? How many times have you taken a new job, moved to a new house, thrown away your old clothes and created a new wardrobe? Well, in a certain sense Earth is going through the same kind of remaking, only on a much grander scale of time. The example I would like to give you is how you birth your own kind. Previously there were no other options for a live birth but for the unborn to come through the birth canal. This is how you are genetically programmed. But now you have created the option of bringing forth the unborn by surgical means. You have also created the possibility of saving the unborn's life at a point in its development that you have labeled "gestational age," a point when no unborn in the past could have survived. And still you devise new ways to re-create, animate in 3-D, and birth yourselves through means that were previously unimaginable. In addition, you are altering your DNA.

As the source of divine nourishment, I hold open three doors for humanity, where previously there was only one way to proceed, on a linear path through time. These doors are opening not sequentially, but simultaneously. This is my threefold gift to you. Through the doorway of your upper chakras, you are connected to the starbeings who look after you. This door is opened by the bees, whom I attract. They open the portal through sound. Through the doorway of your lower charkas, you are connected to the earth and are nourished by my physical medicine. This door is opened by sex and the chemicals that it releases when you are conscious, committed, and connected. The third door is through the portal of your heart, where the upper and lower charkas meet, and it leads to spirit. This magical doorway between the worlds opens when you have completed your earthly karma. It is not dependent on being or not being in physical form, and the key to this door is the surrender of forgiveness. Should you choose to be divinely nourished and walk through these doors into the light of the truth, know that I am holding this light for you as a being who is already in light body, not to simply open your eyes to the truth, but to blind them so that you may see into eternity, for all truths are but half-truths. You will decide how you will be consumed by this life. It is the law of three to be nourished, nurtured, and devoured.

As you make the transition to a New Earth, use my medicine to assist in the transformation of your physical form. The full extent of my medicine is not currently known or fully understood by your scientific communities, but because I have been around for so long and in such great presence, this fact has given me a good laugh. And because I also live in dimensions beyond the limits of the reductionist mind, I was not meant to be fully understood. The only way for you to truly get to know me is by taking enough time so I may nourish you with my wisdom and compassion. I am the source of divine nourishment, in alignment with the Goddess. The act of sex between my flower and the bee goddess serves to harmonize the opposites, but not to unify them, for the loss of diversity is a stress, not unlike the healthy stress of labor that brings forth a new creation. It is a labor of love, and all are in agreement to complete this dance. Mine is a symbol of fertility and abundance.

There is no need to change anyone but yourself. Focus on your own waking consciousness, and remember that the Goddess allows all things. That which you fight against only grows stronger; the struggle is what keeps the wheels of karma spinning. This is your opportunity to step off the wheel into my fields of clover and to be nourished by them. I embody the alchemy of transformation, from soil to flower to bee to golden honey. Why do you think they, the bees, make more than they would ever need? I am pollinating an abundant world for you, my beloveds. I am offering you a field of perception. Walk with me across this field and through the woods and into the meadow clearing. Learn to read my signs as the bees do, through eyes that see polarized light.

Divine nourishment also comes from your relationship with the seasons of birth, life, death, and transformation. It is a cycle with no beginning and no end. Be aware of the cycles of your life, for as you live, so shall you birth, and so shall you die. Just as there is a spring and a rebirth, there is also an autumn and a death. You call the winter of your life the golden years, and indeed they are. But not because of treasures you have hoarded or money you have saved to allow enjoyment of this time, but because of the wisdom you have acquired on your journey through all of life's passages. All of your life is a gift, and even your dying and death are gifts.

Your nourishment on all levels brings me the greatest joy, for this is how you are learning to receive divine love. I, like you, am rooted in the darkness of an old and dying Earth, but together we are opening like a thousand petals to the light of a great and Central Sun. I hold the door open so that you may step from your present world of darkness into the light of a New Earth, for your prayers are my prayers, and it is time to take our birth.

The Tao is called the Great Mother:
empty yet inexhaustible,
it gives birth to infinite worlds.
It is always present within you.
You can use it any way you want.

LAO-TZU

Out beyond ideas of wrongdoing
and rightdoing there is a field.
I'll meet you there.
When the soul lies down in that grass
the world is too full to talk about.

RUMI

Rumi Revisited

What was inanimate became animate
And animate became animal
Animal became human
And human became the being
That must now be leaving
All animal fears of dying
While being called to become something more
With wings and feathers that must also
Be someday laid aside
Along with all the seeking for an angel-god
So as to be even greater than that which had
       to die.

THEA SUMMER DEER

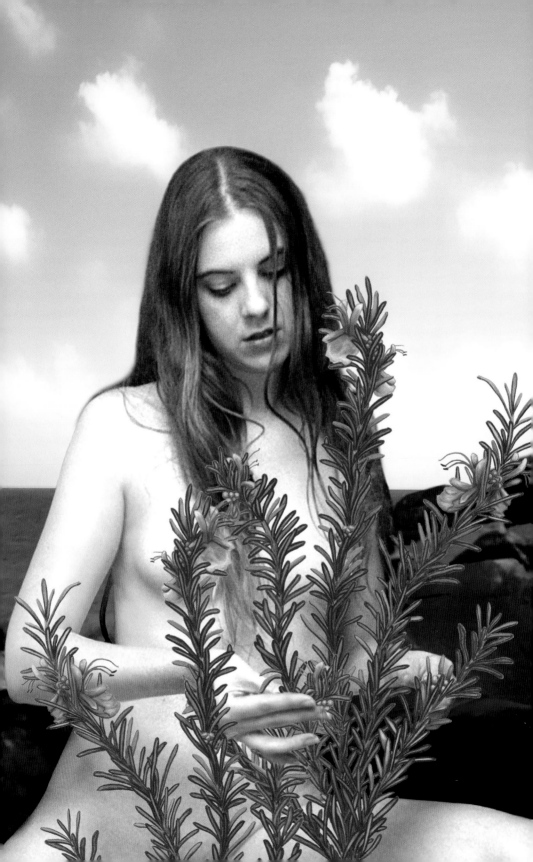

Rosemary

Rosmarinus officinalis

Remembrance

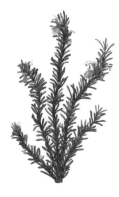 The herb rosemary, *Rosmarinus officinalis,* has been associated with innumerable legends and traditions and put to a hundred uses. A member of the Lamiaceae family, also known as the mint family, rosemary is native to the Mediterranean and one of the most beautiful and fragrant of the culinary herbs. It is aromatic, savory, medicinal, and ceremonial, earning the name "Herb of Remembrance." Because it can tolerate relatively dry growing conditions and has structural features that help it to minimize water loss, rosemary keeps fresh for long periods of time and was used in ancient Egypt as one of the embalming herbs. Rosemary was placed in tombs to remember the dead as far back as the Egyptian First Dynasty, and it is still regarded as a funeral flower, signifying remembrance of the departed.

The dry climate of Egypt contributes to the excellent preservation of organic materials and the ancient secrets that they hold. One of those secrets was discovered in tombs of southern Egypt that date to the fourth century CE. Ancient Egyptian wine jars coated with a residue containing constituents identified as those that could only have come from the herb rosemary reveal

127

one of the most longstanding of ancient traditions: the making of medicinal wines. Numerous vessels with this residue were found littering the ground around taverns in Nubian villages of the period, demonstrating how wine had gone from a beverage of the pharaohs to one of commoners, who were also buried with it.[1]

In Europe as far back as the Middle Ages, rosemary was believed to be offensive to evil spirits and thought to grow only in gardens tended by women pure of heart. So great was the belief in its power that for centuries rosemary was put under pillows at night, hung on walls, strewn on floors, and burned as incense to protect against evil. It has a strong yet delicate pine-like scent that is robust in the upright varieties and less so in the prostrate cultivars, which prefer growing over rocky walls and ledges. Women have also used rosemary since the beginning of time as an abortifacient. If the timing of a pregnancy wasn't right, a woman knew that if she chewed on the fresh leaves and drank an infusion of the sharp, pungent herb, it would cleanse her womb of its contents.

Even though rosemary was used in burial rituals and as a medicine, it was also associated with romantic love and marriage. As a wedding decoration it served as a reminder that even if a couple were leaving friends and family to start a new life, they would never be forgotten. A symbol of fidelity, rosemary was thought to encourage couples to remember their wedding vows and was used in love potions for the purpose of preserving love.

In Greece, rosemary plants are long lived and some grow quite large, up to six feet tall. In one legend, the ancient Greek titaness Mnemosyne, the goddess of memory, met her worshippers at a dark pool and took from them all their earthly memories so they would not suffer in the afterlife. Ancient portraits of Aphrodite show her being draped in rosemary and myrtle by the naiads as she steps out of the ocean and onto the isle of Cypros. Perhaps this is why rosemary is regarded as an aphrodisiac. Modern legends of rosemary are closely associated with the Virgin Mary and Christianity, with Mary's blue cloak thought to be the color of rosemary's flowers. It is also said that a rosemary bush will live for only thirty-three years and grow to be as tall as Christ stood when he was crucified. Legends that have served as the foundation for entire cultures, from the Egyptian myth of the birth of Horus, which begins with his immaculate conception, to rosemary and myrtle being regarded foremost among Mary's plants, still survive today as universal symbols that remind us of our interconnectedness and the continuum of humanity.

THE DIVINATION

If you have called on the spirit of rosemary, you are most likely being asked to remember something, and that "something" may be older than your present religious or familial system. There is great power in remembering, because to hold something in memory is to keep it alive. In a linear progression, where time is seen as continually marching forward, our capacity for retrieving memories is limited and works in only one direction—from the past. In the magical realms, where shamans know how to bend time and walk between the worlds, past, present, and future all exist simultaneously. Emerging sciences like quantum physics are beginning to explore some of these concepts. As our understanding of the workings of the universe continues to evolve, it is important to remain open to new possibilities. One of those possibilities is the ability to remember the past as well as the future, a skill that is encoded in our DNA. There is no going back to the past, but we may continue to recreate more of the same in the future if we do not learn the lessons of our past.

On the spiral journey, which is a portal between linear time and the dimension of illumination, or nonlinear time, we repeat what appears to be the same lessons over and over, only each time at a higher octave, with the memory of everything that has come before informing our present as we move into a future that is not yet in form. Memory is a thought form, and thought precedes matter, or material form. Our physical body, which is material form inhabited by spirit, has its own cellular memory, which is perceived first through the senses. This perception or knowing can be directly experienced at a cellular level. It is through this cellular memory that we activate our DNA and wake up. The spiral path is the bridge between two realities where we are given the opportunity to fully integrate this dimension so that we can move on to the next.

The illumination of matter would not be possible had it not first emerged from the darkness of the void. All matter contains within it a balance of light and dark. If we choose not to climb the evolutionary rungs of the spiral ladder and instead continue to operate with the same limited strands of DNA from our past, then we experience what might be considered a fall from grace. Form returns to formlessness and is rebirthed at an appropriate level of consciousness that serves the continuing evolution of form. From this point of reference, the memory of "the fall" lives in both the future and the past by the same laws that govern this dimension of duality. You cannot have day without night or future without past in this dimension. It is similar to the way a computer does a future projection based on past events, only our minds have the power to manifest those projections in physical, three-dimensional reality. When time ceases to be linear, we will remember our days of future passed and fully enter four-dimensional reality. It is a paradox.

While linear thinking may allow us to comprehend spiral dynamics, a finite mind cannot wrap itself around something that is infinite. The retrieval of memories, both past and future, is necessary for the activation of what was once thought of as our "junk" DNA. It is through this activation that we will evolve into the next dimension of existence and the world of illumination, where we still have bodies, albeit bodies of light. In fact we are already in bodies of light but have not integrated or come into balance with the darkness of our shadow so that we can be fully conscious of who we truly are.

Rosemary is the stimulus that calls on the memories from our past so that we can re-member our future. The ancient Egyptians understood these mysteries and left many clues, including the drinking of rosemary-infused wine and the myth of Isis and Osiris. Past and future live in the portal of the present. We are the future that the Egyptians envisioned in what is now our past. Re-membering takes place in the present moment. It is in the present that we walk between the worlds, get a glimpse of eternity, and awaken to who we are and why we are here. Shame, guilt, remorse, regret, and blame do not exist in nonlinear time. When we step off the path of cause and effect, we become co-creators of a New Earth.

When something is called to memory, its spirit lives in the present. So the question is, What do we want to remember? Most of us would answer that we want to remember things that are positive and life affirming. While traumatic events are also held in memory and must be called back in order to be released and healed, it is the role of rosemary to contact the memories of those things we hold most dear. Rosemary has the ability to open our hearts to the part of us that is childlike and innocent. Allow rosemary to remind you of the power of an open heart and an open mind, for these are the qualities that are necessary at this time.

Rosemary also asks you to remember who is the master of your garden. We are immersed in a patriarchal system that has been supported by the unconscious feminine and that has brought us to the brink of total collapse. We have forgotten what it means to co-create and to live in harmony. Use rosemary in aromatherapy to remember that which you cherish most deeply—the gift of life. When we remember this, we automatically nurture and protect. Rosemary essential oil diluted in olive oil may be used to anoint yourself when going through a shamanic death. If you are in the presence of someone who is getting ready to pass over and that person is open to being anointed, place one drop of the diluted essential oil on each wrist and one on the third eye. This will stimulate spiritual and mental clarity and open a portal through a pyramid of light for a more complete passing, or stepping over, into the next realm. When a life ends—a woman loses her pregnancy for whatever reason, an elder passes on, or anything else departs—branches of rosemary can be placed on the floor and then stepped over as a symbolic way to close the door of the spirit world so that both the living and the dead can move on.

The current system that is passing away from us now was based on fear, domination, and control. Its war cry was "divide and conquer." Ancient knowledge, as held throughout the ages by various secret societies, sages, gurus, and spiritual leaders, has directed us to remember the original instructions given to us by the Creator. These instructions live within every cell of our being.

When an environment becomes extremely polluted, as have our bodies from eating poisoned, depleted, chemically altered, and genetically modified food, it becomes difficult to remember these instructions. Cleanse your mind and your palette with rosemary. Prepare a sacred feast, and set it on your table with a centerpiece of rosemary. Breathe deeply, and let her fragrance awaken your senses to the remembrance of the sacredness of life. Something has given its life so that you may live. Honor it. Season it with rosemary. Plant rosemary at the entrance of your home to impart protection to all who enter and dwell there. Marry it to the magic of the herbs. Preserve it with an open heart.

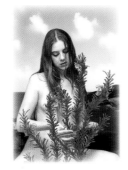

THE DEVA SPEAKS

I have a tale to tell you. It is as old as the oldest tree that grows by the sea, and perhaps it is even older still. It is a story shared mostly among the devas and the nature spirits who near this sea do dwell.

A long, long time ago there lived a man who loved trees. He spent his whole life building sailing ships from wood to sail on the sea. He never took a wife, though he was handsome as a king, but he wanted nothing more than to feel the wood from which he made many a beautiful thing. One day while he was out sailing, a mighty wind came quickly rising and took him with his vessel to the bottom of the deep. The last thing on his mind before his life began to fade was the tall and noble tree from which his sailing ship was made. He asked the spirits of the ocean, he posed the question to the sea, if he were to be born again, might he come back as a tree?

Many years would pass before a maiden walked along the rocky shore. And as she walked she spied a tree so handsome that she fell on her knees. Daily she came to stand before this tall and noble tree, and every day she wished that he could hear her plea. She wished that he could be her lover, wrap his pine bough arms around her, and make love sweetly to her as the wind sang through their hair. She had eyes and arms and hands only for this tree there by the sea, beside which she would stand for hours until the nature spirits took pity on her lovesick reverie.

Now, the deva of the tree forbade this love, but the nature spirits granted her one night in his human company. She came that eve at twilight, for she loved to watch the stars rise behind his handsome silhouette, but what she came to find there, she never would forget. In place of her beloved tree stood a very handsome man, with the darkest hair and greenest eyes that she had ever seen. He looked into her shining eyes of the palest, truest blue and stroked her long and golden flowing hair—there, beside the ocean, lovers now as one, where once there had been two.

A daughter was born of their union, conceived by the nature spirits and forbidden by the deva of the tree. Her given name was Rosmarinus, which means "dew of the sea," and there by the seaside is where she grew. The deva made her not as tall as her father, but her leaves were the green of his eyes and her blossoms spoke of her mother's eyes, the palest, truest blue.

Since the deva had grown angry by this forbidden love, she gave Rosmarinus the power to cause a woman to lose her pregnancy in remembrance of what should never have been. Her seeds are tiny and difficult to propagate, but still she has many offspring, some upright like herself and some who wear their hair of deep green needles draping over the rocky cliffs in remembrance of their mother's long and flowing hair. In her mercy the deva allowed these siblings the power to bring beauty to the earth goddesses, who use rosemary's benefits for their hair and skin.

I tell you this tale so that you may come to understand more deeply the alliance between humans and Rosmarinus, whom you call rosemary, as well as the sympathies of the nature spirits and the responsibilities of the devas. May you honor her medicines as you honor yourselves.

The Rosemary Song

The piney scent of Rosemary
has called your memory near
and brought me to remembrance
of the things I hold most dear

Remember me with Rosemary
where the fog and salt spray meet
for this is where I think of you
upon the isle of Crete

Marry me with Rosemary
I'll wear her flowers pale and blue
and keep you always in my heart
My love for you is true

Bury me with Rosemary
when my time on Earth is through
Toss her there upon my grave
and I will always be with you

THEA SUMMER DEER

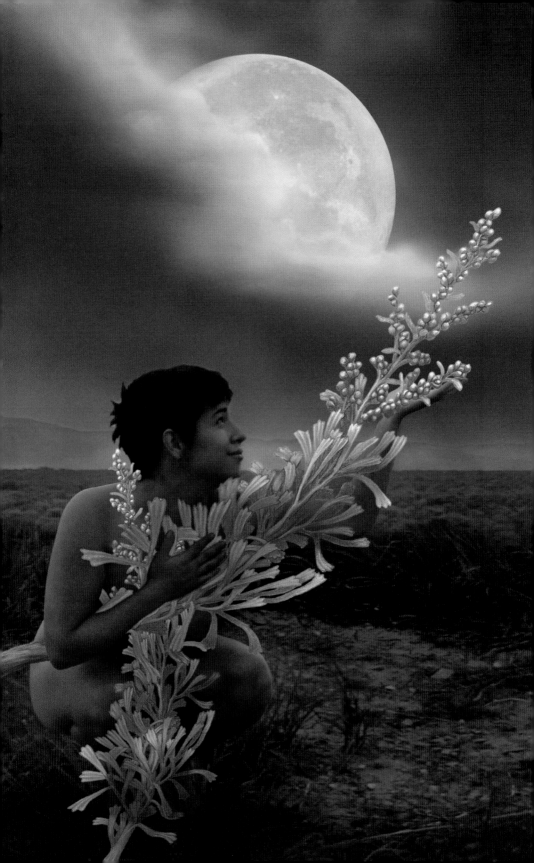

Sagebrush

Artemisia tridentata

Time Keepers

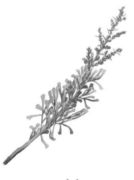

Artemisia tridentata is an elegant name for what is commonly known as sagebrush. The genus *Artemisia* is named after the ancient Greek virgin moon goddess Artemis because its herbs are silver in color and appear to be bathed in moonlight. Artemis was a huntress, healer, and protector of children and women, especially during childbirth. Her consort was a wolf, and like the animals that she hunted and the young girls that she protected, her instincts were intact. To this day, hunters who live or hunt where sagebrush grows cover their scent by rubbing it on their skin and clothes.

The species name, *tridentata,* or "three toothed," describes the three-lobed leaves. *A. tridentata* is in the Asteraceae family and should not be confused with sage, the common name given to many plants of the Lamiaceae family, such as *Salvia officinale,* or garden sage, also known as culinary sage. Other species of *Artemisia* include tarragon (*A. dracunculus*), wormwood (*A. absinthium*), and mugwort (*A. vulgaris*). All are hardy herbs and shrubs known for their aromatic volatile oils. *A. tridentata* is a silvery gray, perennial shrub averaging four feet in height, but there are also several subspecies* that can grow up to fifteen feet. Small wedge-shaped leaves, covered in fine white hairs, typical of plants in the *Artemisia* genus, help minimize water loss. It is found on dry plains, mesas, and rocky areas with deep, well-drained soils, and it grows in vast tracts or more sparsely in cold desert shrub and piñon-juniper woodland habitats.

All of these ecosystems receive an average of eight inches of rain per year, with most precipitation occurring in the winter. Sagebrush is an evergreen, and in late summer, dense clusters of tiny yellow or cream-colored flowers bloom in terminal corymbs,† producing tiny black seeds. Nevada, which is sometimes called the Sagebrush State, has adopted sagebrush as its state flower. The flowers are self-pollinated or wind pollinated, and each plant produces thousands of seeds. Sagebrush, which is not fire resistant, depends on the airborne distribution of its seeds to reestablish itself following wildfires. The wood ignites easily and burns well, making it valuable as a fire starter.

The fragrance of sagebrush when crushed is pleasant and similar to that of culinary sage, but its taste is bitter and unpalatable. The especially strong smell that it gives off after a desert rain can be attributed to the primary constituent of camphor and is thought by botanists to be an adaptation that discourages browsing by ruminants. The leaves have considerable nutritional value for these animals, but the volatile oils are toxic to the symbiotic bacteria necessary for digestion. The only large herbivore to browse sagebrush successfully is the pronghorn antelope, because it evolved alongside sagebrush in one of the most extensive landscapes in North America.‡

Sagebrush grows in the high desert at elevations between four thousand and ten thousand feet and covers over a hundred million acres of the

---

Artemisia tridentata consists of three subspecies: basin big sagebrush (*A. tridentata* ssp. *tridentata*), mountain big sagebrush (*A. tridentata* ssp. *vaseyana*), and Wyoming big sagebrush (*A. tridentata* ssp. *wyomingensis*).

†A corymb is a raceme, or type of inflorescence (flower cluster), in which the stems of the lower flowers are longer than those of the upper flowers so that the inflorescence has a flat-topped appearance overall. This renders the whole inflorescence more conspicuous to insects, and the individual flowers tend to remain small.

‡The pronghorn is not technically an antelope, but it does resemble the true antelopes of the Old World. Due to convergent evolution (the acquisition of the same biological trait in unrelated lineages), it fills a similar ecological niche. All other members of its family, Antilocapridae, are extinct.

American West's romanticized wide-open spaces. This landscape is referred to as the sagebrush steppe, a harsh landscape of subtle beauty and dramatic extremes, where the play of light and shadow is constant and changing. It is characterized by cold, harsh winters and dry summers, where temperatures soar by day and plummet at night. This seemingly endless ocean of sagebrush is home to an amazing variety of high-desert flora and fauna, whose survival depends on the ecosystem. These include black-tailed jackrabbits, pygmy rabbits, pronghorn antelope, collared lizards, sage grouse, Brewer's sparrows, horned larks, prairie falcons, and golden eagles.

There has been some controversy in the environmental conservation community as to the need for preservation of the sagebrush steppe. With the encroachment of civilization, overgrazing by livestock, certain range management practices, and energy development, the sagebrush steppe ecosystem is dwindling. As this occurs, piñon-juniper woodlands, aided by unnatural fire cycles and the invasion of exotic species, are spreading into areas formerly classified as sagebrush steppes.* It wasn't until the 1980s that sagebrush began to be considered a valuable native species rather than a weed. Prior to that, it was routinely chained (a method of removal using a bulldozer and chains), burned, or sprayed with toxic herbicides in an effort to eradicate it. Conservation groups, government agencies, and other stakeholders are still debating whether sagebrush habitat should be restored and how to accomplish this daunting task.

With the invasion of exotic grasses like cheatgrass (*Bromus tectorum*), which are perpetuated through fire and provide a continuous source of fuel that increases the size and frequency of wildfires, coupled with the increased severity of drought, the sagebrush steppe is dying, clearing the way for more cheatgrass in the future. It out-competes native grasses for water and nutrients and thereby "cheats" native fauna species and livestock out of a valuable food source. A monoculture of cheatgrass is not only dominating millions of acres of land but also is changing the soil nutrients, such that invasive grasses are favored over the native plants. Once an area has converted to a monoculture of cheatgrass,

---

*Decades of livestock grazing and fire suppression have created conditions that scientists believe have contributed to the rapid and unnatural spread of western juniper down from the hilltops and across sagebrush basins. Invading juniper, piñon, and pine species thrive in the limited moisture conditions of the sagebrush steppes, which have a high enough elevation to encourage it.

it has little chance of recovery. Wildlife species that depend on the sagebrush steppe are experiencing a steep decline in their populations because of this habitat loss. Sagebrush steppe habitats are essential for the survival of pronghorn and sage grouse; both are endangered species and uniquely adapted to consume sagebrush.

The pronghorn's struggle is multiplied due to habitat fragmentation, sheep and cattle ranchers' fences, and shrinking migration corridors. In the United States, the attempts to fence, monitor, and secure the border with Mexico by the Department of Homeland Security are seen as a hindrance in efforts to save the Sonoran pronghorn by environmentalists and the U.S. Fish and Wildlife Service.* Pronghorns are the fastest land mammals in North America, crossing large tracts of land at high speed, but they are not good at jumping fences. Their meat is very desirable, and they are widely hunted by humans and less successfully by predators.

The sage grouse is another icon of the Wild West on the sagebrush steppe, and it is the largest grouse in North America. Settlers called them sage chickens and ate them along with domestic poultry. The Gunnison sage grouse is also an endangered species dependent on the sagebrush ecosystem.† It uses sagebrush for its mating dance and nesting cover, and has a diet consisting of mostly sagebrush foliage and buds, with this being its only food source throughout the winter. The Audubon Society lists the Gunnison sage grouse as one of the ten most endangered birds in North America. It is only through the preservation of habitat that these species will survive, but loss of habitat and the resulting loss of fauna is not a new story in an ever-changing landscape on the shifting sands of time.

American Indians living in the desert southwest have always had a close relationship with sagebrush, collecting it as firewood and using it in building construction. Sagebrush is also used externally as a natural insect repellent and shows promise as a nontoxic fumigant for grain storage facilities. The Navajo and Hopi use it medicinally to rid the body of parasites. The

---

*The Sonoran pronghorn is a subspecies that lives in Mexico and Arizona. It has been protected under the Endangered Species Act since 1967.
†The Gunnison sage grouse was newly named in 2000 for Gunnison, Colorado, where it lives high up in the mountains.

Artemesias have long been known for this use, giving rise to their other common name, wormwood. The Navajo and Hopi also used sagebrush internally to stop hemorrhaging and to treat infections. The Ute used the shredded bark for candlewicks, wove its fibers into footwear and clothing, and made sacks of the woven bark and lined them with native grasses. Navajo weavers boiled the leaves and flowers to create a golden dye for their wool. In the sagebrush hills when a Navajo baby is born, he or she is seen as belonging to the clan of the mother, and one of these clans is the Sagebrush Hill Clan.

In northern New Mexico, where the sage-covered hills seem to roll endlessly toward the horizon, sagebrush is known as *chamiso pardo,* or gray sagebrush, and the tea is used to treat many conditions, from colds, coughs, flu, toothaches, and arthritis to digestive problems.

Indigenous knowledge and use of sagebrush is supported by medical research, which attributes many of sagebrush's medical actions to the chemical constituents of its volatile oils, specifically the monoterpene identified as camphor. Camphor, most often harvested from the camphor tree, *Cinnamomum camphora,* or synthetically produced, is used medicinally in several commercial preparations as a cough suppressant and as a topical analgesic. As a rubefacient for external application, camphor increases circulation and acts as a counterirritant to reduce joint inflammation and heal muscle sprains. Readily absorbed through the skin, camphor is cooling, mildly anesthetic, and antimicrobial. When we use the whole of sagebrush medicinally, rather than an isolated volatile oil or a synthetic reproduction, we get the benefit of the plant's synergy, which has been time tested in remedies and preparations of teas and infusions for internal and external use. Sagebrush, however, should be used with caution as a medicine. Sensitive individuals may contract allergic dermatitis after contact with sagebrush. Because sagebrush contains high amounts of volatile oils, large doses may be toxic.

Steam-distilled sagebrush essential oil is complex and rich in terpenoids, which contribute to its scent, primarily that of camphor. The interest in therapeutic applications of essential oils is steadily increasing as people continue the search for alternative ways to improve their health, yet the chemical composition and effect of many of these oils are still unknown. This is surprising in light of the evidence that when inhaled through aromatherapy or applied directly to the skin, essential oils affect the autonomic nervous system, enter the bloodstream, and act like a drug. Because the essential oil of *A. tridentata* contains toxic chemical components, it should be regarded as potentially hazardous.*

Camphor is the most active chemical compound found in sagebrush, and the use of camphor as a healing agent varies among traditions. For example, in Ayurvedic medicine, the ancient East Indian system of healing, it is considered an antibacterial agent. In traditional Chinese medicine, it is used to strengthen and activate the nervous system and stimulate digestion. In Africa, the bark has been used to reduce fever, treat malaria, and as a general antiseptic. In addition to its uses as a medicine, camphor is also an important ceremonial agent. In India, camphor is used in incense to clarify the mind. In Hindu pujas and ceremonies, it is burned in a holy flame celebrating Shiva, the god of destruction and re-creation. Because camphor contains a natural pitch that burns cool without leaving an ash residue, it is seen as a symbol for pure consciousness.

Sagebrush is a sacred herb that has been used for generations by Native American peoples throughout the Southwest for spiritual cleansing, much the same way that camphor is burned in India. Cleansing people, places, and objects by smudging with the smoke of burning herbs and resins is an ancient practice. This method was also used to repel insects and preserve food and animal hides. In some traditional Native American medicine practices, it is used in smudging ceremonies to clear negative energy from an individual or environment. Sagebrush is also included in pouches and bundles for protection. Native American medicine men and women teach that wherever sage is burned, negative entities cannot enter or occupy the same space and must leave.† In the Lakota *Inipi* (sweat lodge) ceremony, sage is brought into the lodge and placed on the hot rocks, where it releases its fragrant smoke and purifying essence.

The flower essence of sagebrush is a valuable energetic medicine used for clearing obstacles, illusions, and habitual patterns from one's physical, men-

---

*The primary constituents of *A. tridentata* essential oil are camphor, camphene, cineole, and a small amount of thujone. Thujone may cause convulsions and fatty degeneration of the liver, while camphene is regarded as nontoxic, nonirritating, and nonsensitizing. Cineole is safe in the amounts found in an essential oil, but if ingested can cause poisoning and gastrointestinal and central nervous system damage.

†Unrelated to sagebrush, white sage, *Salvia apiana,* is also used as a sacred herb in this way.

tal, emotional, and spiritual bodies. It can increase awareness of the places where our lives are stuck and help us release attachments to addictions and self-destructive habits. Of particular value is sagebrush's ability as a flower essence to help one discover a new self-identity when the old one falls away. It assists with the entire process of self-realization: the breakthrough, release, transformation, rebirth, and integration of a new spiritual self. Sagebrush, whether used for smudging or as a flower essence, is an agent for the purification and transformation of heart, mind, and body.

THE DIVINATION

If the Medicine Wheel Garden turns and the point of entry is not clear, look within yourself and see what needs to shift. Then open your eyes to the light-filled sky as you find yourself standing at the edge of time. The Time Keepers are not clocks, watches, or calendars, but members of an ancient culture, a plant community of sagebrush that has been evolving on Earth for over five million years.* If you have called on the medicine of sagebrush, then you are ready to embark on a journey into the great unknown across the mesa seas of sage. All rites of passage and times of transformation require purification. To leave what is known to create something new, something must die. Death itself is a time of transition and uncertainty, and the way needs to be made clear for a safe passage. This clearing and purification comes with the aid of the Time Keepers, who hold in their cellular structure the memory of all that has transpired: the deaths and rebirths in the dimension of linear time and space, the unfolding and the calling back into the fold.

The burning of sagebrush renders its physical entity into spiritual form, and this plant acts as a mediator between the physical and spiritual realms. The cleansing breath of smoke is sweet to the spirits who walk the river of stars known as the Milky Road, across the shifting winds of time. It sends a message into the ether of our purified intent and calls the spirits to be with us as much-needed guides.

Time as we know it is an illusion. As we fly out toward the horizon, toward the dividing line of earth and sky, we are flying into time. Time is capable of expanding and collapsing, and the more accelerated our journey

---

*Researchers studying ancient pollen samples believe that the genus *Artemisia* evolved in Eurasia. Mountain big sagebrush (*Artemisia tridentata* ssp. *vaseyana*), the most genetically primitive form, evolved during the middle Pliocene epoch, which began approximately five million years ago.

becomes, the more we can see that it is part of a great multidimensional web. We can view this web through projection and mirroring. Just as we project three-dimensional objects onto two-dimensional surfaces and create the illusion of 3-D, our consciousness is projected into the fourth dimension and mirrored back to us in the illusion of the third dimension.

Religions are born from this kind of projecting, when in essence we are the mirrors of the gods and goddesses that have been projected into the fourth dimension. In a like manner, we are viewing the fourth dimension from the third dimension by projecting time onto space, which creates the illusion of time in 3-D. These other planes of existence exist simultaneously and are being mirrored back to us in 3-D. Crop circles are one example of how the higher dimensions of unconditional love and sacred geometry are being both mirrored and projected into the third dimension. The opening of portals by events such as flying into the horizon, stepping into the energetic field of a crop circle, and standing in a vortex or on a spiral mound used for teleportation, such as those created by the Anasazi, can potentially take us out of this dimension and into nonlinear space and time.

The reality of circular time is something known and embraced by shamans, ancients, and indigenous cultures throughout our history. They knew that all projection is illusion and were able to journey and work with the shadow in order to transmute it. As we move into alignment with the galactic center, the light of a Central Sun illuminates the human psyche, much the same way as when we shine a light on a three-dimensional object and a two-dimensional shadow is cast. The shadows of the human psyche caused by this illumination are being brought to our awareness, giving us an opportunity for integration not previously available during the age of ego-driven fear. Integration of the shadow occurs when we own our projections. By entering nonordinary reality in nonlinear time, we can begin to "see" and identify these projections as they become mirrored in our three-dimensional reality. This kind of journeying into nonordinary reality is aided by the cleansing smoke of the Time Keepers, who are guardians of the portals between these dimensions.

As long as we use logic to figure out the how and why of our journeys and lives, the potential exists for getting stuck in linear time. When we learn to see life as a gestalt and as existing within cycles of time, then we will begin to feel more at ease on our journey and less enamored of the projections. Surrendering to the great unknown is our biggest challenge. Not giving it up to a higher external power, but being in our own higher power. Not absorbing, but emanating. In the past, this kind of power was identified with ego, but we now have systems of healing that overlap, and these are giving us a bigger picture of who we are and who we are becoming. The fear-driven ego was only a part of our spiritual development and integration.

The continuum of space and time is our current definition of the fourth dimension, with time being the final mystery that will take us into the higher dimensions. In *Hamlet,* Shakespeare said, ". . . time is out of joint." What we see occurring in the world today are different time zones, not in geographical terms but represented by different people living at different times of our history. Literacy, for example, was only recently obtained in certain cultures but has existed in others for a much longer period of time. This is true in many areas of human development, such as equality for women and standards of living. What is different today is that the space-time continuum has sped up to the point where cultures that took thousands of years to acquire a single skill or technology are acquiring multiple technologies all at once.

This rapid acquiring of skill and technology has expanded our perception, and we now know that this world is not solid, it only seems that way. Dense vibrational fields appear as solid physical objects, but spiritual essence appears and disappears, and shape shifts from one state to another. Multidimensional frequencies are continually being broadcast into this reality, as evidenced by crop circles, but we have only tuned in the one that we call space and linear time. Since this is the frequency that we hold in our current physical form, it in turn becomes the frequency that we broadcast back into the space-time continuum. When we tune in the fifth dimension, the next four dimensional realities will open up to us.

We are at a crossroads described by the Hopi as the end of the Fourth World of separation and the beginning of the Fifth World of illumination. As physical beings living in the Fourth World of separation, or the fourth dimension, considered by some to be the first dimension of time, we have boundaries as to what we can perceive through our current physical form. Our evolving consciousness, however, is capable of perceiving beyond these imposed limits and into the Fifth World of illumination. It is from this world that the deva of sagebrush speaks to us. One of the ways we can glimpse the movement of consciousness into the next dimension is through the perception that we are living in a unified field. The distance between things in space is not so great the farther out you go. Time creates the illusion that everything is separate.

Everything emits a frequency, has a spirit, and is connected to the web within a unified field of evolving consciousness that is constantly moving. We have previously known only the movement of matter through the physical plane, but more and more we are beginning to perceive the movement of spirit through the ether. As we realize our interconnectedness—that we all breathe the same air, drink the same water, and are made of the same earth—we become self-realized. Self-realization, or self-awareness, is an integrated state of being that shifts and defines our consciousness and broadens our horizons. The vehicle of our light body is expanding into other dimensions at the same time that our physical world appears to be collapsing. It is right and perfect, as matter can neither be created nor destroyed; it simply goes through a transformation and changes form.

We are literally moving through the dimensions of space and time into timelessness and infinite space, but we cannot perceive something infinite with something finite. Only by surrendering the mind and entering the dreamtime can we begin to glimpse what is possible beyond the limits of time and space. In the dreamtime we can view and move through other dimensions in ways not possible in our waking reality. In the dreamtime it is possible to be two places at the same time. The Time Keepers are dimensional portals. By clearing the way into the unknown with the aid of sagebrush, which has been holding this space for millennia, we will be assured a safe passage. This medicine cannot be underestimated, for it is of tremendous spiritual value at this time.

The instinctual nature represented in the goddess Artemis knows the appropriate time for all things: time to let live what is yet to come, time to let die what is past, time to act, time to rest, time to make love, time to be alone. The old cliché "timing is everything" could not be more true. The Time Keepers are the ancestors who lived this knowledge. Just as you might patiently wait for a child to grow to the point of being able to take care of himself or herself, sagebrush knew how long it would take to hold space for the shift we are about to make. The experiences of the collective, instinctual self are encoded in our DNA. Sagebrush remembers over five million years of planetary evolution: the burning, the regeneration, seeds carried on the wind, the vast expanses of space and time that it has occupied. We can remember too, all the way back to the beginning of time, through the ancestors from whom we have taken our birth, and even before that. Not only is it written in the stars and encoded in the stories passed down to us through the generations, but it also lives in each and every cell of our being.

There is a reason why our instinctual self has been historically repressed. This has taken place so that we could be more easily manipulated and controlled. We were told that only animals have instincts, and we were methodically persecuted for using our free will. Because information can be twisted, it has become essential that we develop our intuitive and emotional faculties, as we can no longer rely on just our logical abilities to accurately interpret the information that is being fed to us. Woven within the phases of the human lifetime—infant, child, adolescent, adult, and elder—is the knowledge of the instinctual self. The instinctual self knows what is needed in any given moment and knows that we always have everything we need. This instinctual self is the closest to our soul, and the right use of will comes when we are in alignment with our soul.

The map of time is written in the landscape of our ancestral codes, and time, as we know it, is ending. To access this map we have only to shift our perception from what we think we know to the great unknown, the source of insight and intuition. Through this shift our world will be transformed. When we enter nonordinary reality, time as we know it becomes suspended. It is a kind of *bardo,* or in-between place, where we experience time out of time. It is an evolved consciousness space where great synchronicities occur.

We are learning to become time travelers, and we are crossing time zones at speeds that were incomprehensible less than two generations ago. As our bodies traverse time and distance, we are also crossing ancestral lands. The spirits of these ancestors are holding the above and below energies of earth and sky in that particular space where they lived and died. It is important to remember that we are crossing sacred ground and to request permission to enter, cross, or fly through these energy vortexes. One way to do this is with the sacred smoke of sagebrush. Use it to contact the ancestors and to send them prayers of respect and gratitude. This will clear the path. You could also tuck a sprig of sage on your person or in your travel bag while being aware of where you are and what vortexes you are traveling through.

The effect that time travel is having on our nervous system is tremendous. We are evolving at an increasingly accelerated rate. Past and future are merging in the ever-present now. While we are still in a body, making a journey that we can map in coordinates of space-time, accelerated as it may be, our consciousness is expanding into nonordinary time. The Time Keepers not only show us the route into this alternate reality through the cloak of their cleansing smoke, but they also help us to release the spiritual essence of our ethereal bodies so we can make the journey without becoming fragmented. We are shifting into light body. Sagebrush has been taking in more light for a longer period of time than any other medicine presently available to us.

Multidimensional awareness is simply the knowledge that we are not separate from All That Is. This knowledge takes place in the presence of expanding light, is accompanied by sound, and can be accessed through the breath. It is an experience where the divisions between matter and spirit, and even life and death, are reconciled and returned to source as matter becomes infused with spiritual light. In this experience we taste the divine nectar that flows through our physical bodies directly from our soul and connects us with the light beings of the devic world, who are holding the door open for our transformation. This is spiritual knowledge of the drop of water returning to the ocean of consciousness that holds and expresses our connection to the infinite and the divine. In truth, we have always been a part of this great ocean. Open your eyes, for the sagebrush sea is awash with the radiant light of a new dawning of consciousness. Know that the way has been made clear and safe for your journey toward the horizon of a New Earth.

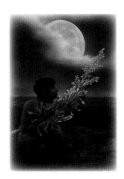

THE DEVA SPEAKS

So you want to go beyond the boundaries of space and time? It is a vast illusion, this thing that you call time. And for so long you have created all of your reference points within it. You feel trapped by having either too much or not enough, and you use old metaphors like "time is money," which indeed it is. No one can give you more time or take it away from you. Only you can give it to yourself and allow yourself or others to take it from you. If you feel that you don't have enough time because you are constantly stuffing yourself full of things to do, then you may want to look at what drives this kind of greed. It is not a negative thing, but a necessary phase of transformation to consume the world before entering the chrysalis. And as you enter the chrysalis, surrender all thought of emergence, for nothing should interfere with this time that requires nothing less than complete dissolution of form.

You must give up everything you know to become something wholly new. Be mindful of this in your consumption. What experiences do you value the most? Some of you believe that the short time you are alive on the earth in a physical body is the only time you have. But I am here in my present and eternal form as the Keeper of Time to tell you: the source of the records of time is soon to be revealed.

If you really want to get to know yourself in time, so that you can learn to journey out of time, then take yourself on a vacation. Put away your watch, computer, calendar, and cell phone. Rise with the sun. Eat when you are hungry. Watch the sunset, and go to sleep when you are tired. Reflect on the ever-changing light, the dance of shadows, and the heavenly stars at night. See how long it takes you to forget what day it is and discover the irrelevance of time. Remember to breathe deeply, go for walks, and swim in the river. Does the thought of doing this make you uncomfortable, or does it make you long for more simplicity? To what have you given your time, and how great is the price you have paid? For what have you traded your time? For what are you saving up more time? Do you remember how when you were a child your world was timeless? I am here to assist you on your journey in time and out of time so that you can experience the magic of living in synchronistic time.

The common belief that, given enough time, our hurts will heal is an illusion, but this way of thinking has kept you in denial. It is possible to heal spontaneously in an instant, because all time exists simultaneously on different frequencies. You are about to experience a renaissance of consciousness in which instead of aspiring to move at the speed of light, you will learn to travel at the speed of thought.

Layers of time, like when you look into the geological layers of the Grand Canyon carved out by the rivers of time, will reveal secrets from your ancient past. The stories that you tell yourselves over and over are what carve out your well-worn reality, but when the earth relinquishes her hidden secrets, you will learn a new and different history of yourselves.

Many of your scientists have become concerned about "threshold effects," and they believe that once a threshold is crossed, there will be no going back. While it may seem that the system in which I have evolved is reaching a certain threshold in which invasive native and nonnative species are taking over, or "invading my space," I assure you that it is all part of the natural plan.

I have lived for a long time and have seen many things, and I would ask that you not be overly concerned with the extinction of species. This may shock you, and while it pulls on your heartstrings and you grieve deeply for what has been and is being lost, the time is coming when your species will go by the same road as your companions. For there was a time before you were created and there will be a time after you are destroyed, according to the laws of your dimension. What lies beyond your temporal world of physical form and matter lives in the realm of the ether.

Your world will not end. It will be transformed. Breathe in to this, for it is toward this world that you are evolving. Your breath doesn't stop from the first breath to the last. The pump of creation, breathing in and breathing out, maintains the world with positive and negative ions. All of life in the universe is pulsating with this same breath, including your solar sun. You and I are inextricably linked through this breath. My exhale is your inhale, and together we co-create this and many other worlds. Allow me to share with you a little story about my ancestors, a long-lived people who sailed across the Mesa Sea to the shores of a new world.

Throughout time, as you may know, many tribes of people gathered where my boughs of sagebrush grow. In one such time, very long ago, before the seas subsided, a tribe of children agreed to be my future keeper. They made a contract of the soul, which was very wide and deep, so as to include that when their contract was complete they would not die, but would simply turn and swim away to yet another sea. These Children of the Earth lived long on the Mesa Sea, and as the earth was shifting, they gave birth to me.

By way of the evening star they came, shining brightly with her love, and became a living library from the shining stars above. They dug their houses into the earth, where they lived and danced, and sang and prayed, beneath the stars from which they came. When from the kiva they emerged, they shared the songs that they had learned. These songs held the secrets of the earth, and they were passed down to all the children that they birthed. Passed down to me. This knowledge was shared through story and rhyme, and set sail on the ocean of time. An oral tradition, echoing down the canyon walls on the vibration of sound, telling us how all living beings are related to All That Is and disclosing all the ancient stories of the healing medicines. They shared with their children's children's children a deeper understanding of what it is to be human in a time of physical and spiritual fragmentation. The Children of the Earth created something whole in their past and present form, through which something broken in the future could be restored. They knew that they were linked to our future, as surely as we are to their past. The reference points would change, but the connection would always last. And no matter how destructive future generations may become, the Children of the Earth remember who we are and tell the greater story of our home among the stars. They are the record keepers now swimming in the deep, and I, the Keeper of Time, became the Sagebrush Sea. Listen, the earth again is shifting, and you can hear my song if you put your heart against the ground. Like my ancestors before me, I will make my way, back to the motherland that lies beneath the waves. The way has been charted through a course of blood and bone, bringing and carrying and calling us back, singing us back home.

So come and gather the ancient wisdom from my branches, pollinated on the winds of time, for I am a wise old sage. Gather me to cleanse your thoughts and purify your heart. I will speak to you of wide open spaces and endless time. Let your spirit ride unfettered and free out onto the high plains and across the sagebrush sea. Gather my medicine for your journey across the expanse of space and time into the great unknown. Nothing is ever lost in time; it only changes form.

> *She would find them, going west, flanked by ghosts, accompanied by her beloved dead, by fallen heras and heroes and villains and the ranks of the moon and the evening*

star, west against the bright slanting rays of the sun and the turning clock of earth, until west became east, until sunset became sunrise, until time swallowed its own tail and the day that was ending became a day that just beginning to dawn.

STARHAWK

Rainbow Song

Yes there was a rainbow
But you were sleeping at the time
And tomorrow there'll be a rainbow
If you're not sleeping at that time

Yes there was a sunrise
But you were sleeping at the time
And tomorrow there'll be a sunrise
If you're not sleeping at that time

Time, time . . .

Yes there are some flowers
Growing out of the altar of time
And tomorrow smell those flowers
If you're not sleeping at the time

Yes I know there are hungry people
I know they're thirsty all the time
And tomorrow they'll still be thirsty
Saving up more time

Take these drops of water
Let them wash away history and time
But tomorrow there'll be a rainbow
As we dance along through time

Through time, time, through time, time . . .

SANANDA RA

Let Us Ride

Let me ride . . .
Upon your back
Open your wings
And never look back
Into the wide . . .
Open space
Let us ride

Let me ride . . .
Upon your back
Onto the trails
And never look back
Out on the wide . . .
Open range
Let us ride

Let me ride . . .
Upon your back
Into the sea
And never look back
Deep into the wide . . .
Open blue
Let us ride

Let us ride . . .
Into our hearts
Open up wide
And never go back
Into the wide . . .
Great unknown
Let us ride

SANANDA RA

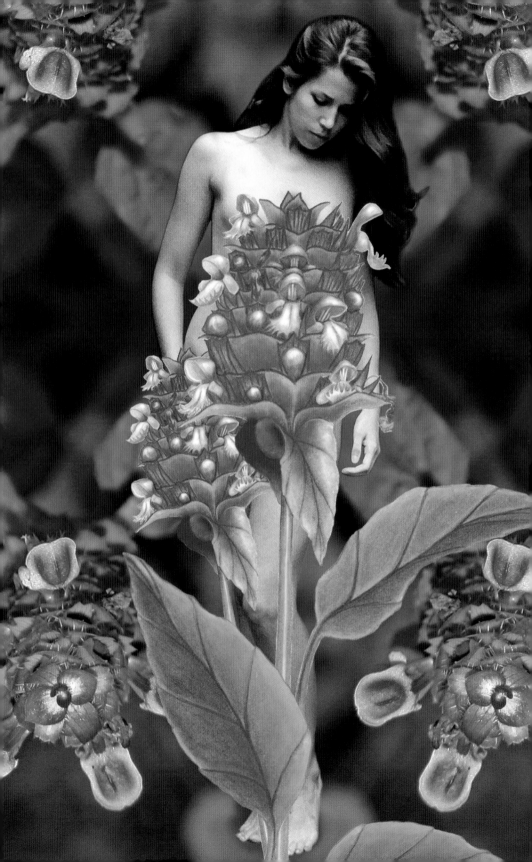

Self-Heal

Prunella vulgaris

....

Unconditional Self-Love

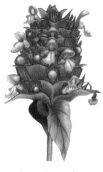

While the name Prunella may elicit the image of a prissy princess or call to mind an Italian folktale,[1] *Prunella vulgaris* is a common perennial wildflower. The genus includes seven species that are all known by the common name self-heal. Self-heal has been used medicinally for centuries on practically every continent to treat just about every ailment. The Latin name *Prunella* means "little prune" and may be derived from the French word *brunelle,* meaning "little plum." Perhaps it is *Prunella's* little purple flowers that cause its association with little plums and prunes. The Latin species name, *vulgaris,* was used by Linnaeus in his naming of plants to describe weedy plants that were common in the landscape. *Vulgaris* means "common" or "ordinary," and when used to refer to people, means "belonging to the ordinary class."

But this word did not always mean vulgar or common. Prior to the European Renaissance, the common people throughout the British Isles used a different form of the word *vulgaris* or *vulgar* to mean "abundance," "sufficiency," or "enough."*

---

*The Celtic word *gwal'ch* means "abundance," and the related word *gwala* means "sufficiency, enough."

Other folk names for this unassuming herb include heal all and heart-of-the-earth, both referring to this plant's ability to heal all wounds internal and external.

A slightly bitter member of the square-stemmed Lamiaceae family of mints, self-heal doesn't have the aromatic qualities usually associated with this family. Its little purple flowers have a hooded upper lip and a fringed lower lip, and they are arranged in whorls at the terminal end of an upright stem. Self-heal blooms constantly from May to September.

Self-heal is a medicinal plant (or a weed, some would say) that is incredibly abundant and found practically all over the world. It grows in the temperate to arctic portions of North America, Europe, Asia, and North Africa. This ecozone, referred to as Holarctic, is a very large region with shared geographical influences. These influences help to explain why plants common to the southern Appalachians are also native to northern parts of eastern Asia. The botanical term for this is *plant disjunction*. Some flora native to the Holarctic ecozone are remnants of a contiguous forest that extended across the northern land masses into what are now the mountains of northern China. As a result, self-heal is part of the materia medica of traditional Chinese medicine and European folk medicine. After the plant spread into North America, it was incorporated into American Indian and Appalachian folk medicine.

Self-heal has a long history of folk use, especially in the treatment of wounds. Prior to World War II, it was used to staunch bleeding and treat heart disease. Considered one of the faery herbs in rural Ireland, perhaps because of its wand of delicate purple flowers and ability to heal, it inspired the young English artist Cicely Mary Barker (1895–1973). In one of her famous flower illustrations, she depicted the self-heal faery as a tiny Florence Nightingale who tends to the injuries of her fellow faeries and little woodland creatures. Cicely Mary Barker's art elicited a sense of freedom of spirit that charmed a war-weary world in the early twentieth century with a vision of innocence and hope. She wrote the following poem to accompany the self-heal faery illustration.

The Song of the Self Heal Faery

When little Elves have cut themselves,
Or Mouse has hurt her tail,

Or Froggies arm has come to harm,
This herb will never fail.
The Faeries skill can cure each ill
And soothe the sorest pain;
She'll bathe and bind,
and soon they'll find
That they are well again.

CICELY MARY BARKER

The seventeenth-century English botanist, herbalist, physician, and astrologer Nicholas Culpeper wrote that this plant is called self-heal because, "When you are hurt, you may heal yourself."[2] According to the Doctrine of Signatures, used by herbalists during the same period, self-heal flowers were thought to resemble the shape of a mouth and were used extensively as a leaf tea to treat sore throats and mouth sores.*

Self-heal grows easily in any damp soil with a pH that is basic or neutral, in full sun or in light shade. Only the aerial parts of the plant, either fresh or dried, are used in herbal medicine. For fresh use self-heal is best harvested early in the season, when the shoots and leaves are still tender, and for drying it is best picked in midsummer, while still in flower. The flowers provide nectar for a multitude of butterflies and bees, and the plant is a beneficial host for the clouded sulphur butterfly. Normally, the plant grows from seed in the spring, but it will also propagate through root division.

The herbal actions of self-heal are so many that it is usually considered to

---

*The Doctrine of Signatures is a spiritual philosophy in which the hand of a higher power (God) was thought to mark everything with a sign, and the sign indicated what the creation could be used for. Because self-heal flowers resemble a mouth, for instance, they would be used to treat problems associated with the mouth. The popularity of this philosophy was aided by Jacob Boehme's book *The Signature of All Things*, published in the first half of the seventeenth century. The Doctrine of Signatures led to the concept of astrological influence, put forward by Nicolas Culpeper. Culpeper felt that only astrologers were fit to study medicine. He then published a translation of the London dispensary medical text from the Latin into the vernacular so that common people could wean themselves from dependency on doctors and delve into the mysteries that were formerly known only to trained physicians.

be an herbal panacea. Self-heal is high in rosmarinic acid, more than rosemary itself, and it is used as an antimicrobial, anti-inflammatory, and antioxidant. In addition, self-heal also exhibits the following herbal actions: alterative, antimutagenic, antispasmodic, astringent, carminative, diuretic, febrifuge, hypotensive, immunostimulant, stomachic, styptic, vermifuge, vulnerary, and tonic. (Please see the section on Herbal Actions in the back of this book for an explanation of these terms.) It is used to gradually restore health, promote wound healing, stop internal hemorrhaging by contracting blood vessels, reduce fever, cause tissues to contract, relieve symptoms of indigestion such as hyperacidity and gas, strengthen and tone the stomach, treat edema, induce urination, lower blood pressure, and even expel intestinal worms. An old French proverb, popularized by Reullius,* states, "No one wants a surgeon who keeps Prunelle."

Fresh picked self-heal can be used to create an herbal poultice and applied directly to a wound. Although it is most commonly used topically to treat sores, burns, and bruises, it is also used internally to relieve hemorrhaging, fevers, diarrhea, and swollen glands. In Chinese medicine, self-heal is classified as cooling to the liver and is used to treat liver and gallbladder inflammation and stagnation. Clinical studies indicate that self-heal inhibits the growth of a number of bacterial infections. These studies have increased interest in this plant's antimicrobial activity and its use as an effective antibiotic for the treatment, both internally and externally, of chronic ulcerations, slow-healing wounds, and other infectious conditions. There is also evidence to support the traditional use of self-heal in the treatment of some forms of cancer, as well as type 2 diabetes. Its antiviral actions seem to slow cell division, making it a potential aid in the treatment of HIV and disease associated with the herpes simplex virus.

Although self-heal is found abundantly in wastelands where the soil has been disturbed, there is nothing wasteful about this plant. Both edible and medicinal, the leaves can be made into a cold-water infusion and drank as a refreshing beverage or made into a hot-water infusion and drank

---

*Ruellius studied medicine, became a doctor in 1508, and was elevated to physician to Francis I in 1509. Ruellius made some of the earliest attempts to popularize botany, as evidenced in his elegantly written *De natura stirpium* (Paris, 1536).

as a tea. The leaves can be eaten as a salad green or cooked in soups and stews. Care should be taken, however, to first thoroughly wash the leaves to remove some of the bitter tannins. Listed as an invasive species with the Center for Invasive Species and Ecosystem Health, self-heal is especially fond of lawns that have not been treated with a weed killer. It epitomizes the popular gardener's quote, "May all your weeds be wildflowers." Since *weed* is a concept created by people and not by nature, we would do well to ask, as did Ralph Waldo Emerson, "What is a weed? A plant whose virtues have not yet been discovered."[3]

THE DIVINATION

A certain plant is trying very hard to get our attention, and she is called self-heal. When the faery princess of the Medicine Wheel Garden appears, it is time to wake up, have a look around, and realize that we have been walking on our medicine. She has made herself very available, and it is no coincidence that she grows most readily where human hands and machines have disturbed the soil.

Self-heal wants us to heal, and she has brought herself into close proximity, and relationship, with humans for this reason. This is the medicine that is needed at this time. She cools our livers, heals our anger, and teaches us how to heal and love ourselves unconditionally. Love is the greatest healer, and this plant loves us so much that she just keeps showing up—practically everywhere! Sometimes, when people have been badly damaged or wounded through neglect or violence, we have to love them until they are able to love themselves. This is what the devas of the medicine plants are doing—loving us until we learn how to love ourselves. Take a moment to look around. Where is this plant growing near you? How will you honor her medicines? There is no imbalance that she cannot restore. You have only to open your heart and receive.

"Love thy neighbor as thyself" implies that one must start by learning to love oneself. If we look around at our neighbors in the world today, we can see that we have not done so well with this lesson. Why is it so difficult to truly love oneself? Perhaps it is because of what we were taught about being born.

Were we born in blessing or born in sin? How were we raised? Were we loved and supported and encouraged to carry our gifts, or were we told that we were bad and punished? Perhaps it is because we have become disconnected from our source, the essence of who we truly are as human beings, dependent on the Earth Mother for our sustenance and for our healing. Perhaps it is because of the pain and suffering we have experienced from this disconnection and the resulting soul loss, for how can we love a self that is not fully present?

When we love ourselves enough to do the inner work of bringing back our lost soul pieces, whose absence keeps us from being fully present, and we integrate those pieces into our three-dimensional physical form, then we free ourselves, and others, to experience new levels of consciousness. We become present in love. Since we live in a holographic universe, when we proclaim to love our self, we proclaim our love for all things. Reclaiming these disenfranchised parts of ourselves is powerful soul work. This work can be accomplished only when we become willing to journey into our shadow, our unconscious, and embrace our own inner darkness. It is a journey where we die to our past ego self and are reborn in what we may call unconditional love—a love that has no reason, a love we share without understanding.

Self-heal brings us a message of innocence and hope in a war-weary world, much the same way that Cicely Mary Barker did with her flower faeries. Self-heal waves her delicate purple wand and beckons us to come closer. She is a common herb for the common people. Never underestimate the common people as a force for transformation. It is through our commonality, our sharing and belonging to the community as a whole, that social change is born. We are in need of such a change and are in the throes of such a birth. The power of self-heal is the power of the people to heal all on levels. We are at the end of a great age, where the love of power is dying, and at the beginning of a new age, where the power of love is rising—rising from the very ground of our being. With this power, the power of unconditional love, the sky is the limit.

We now have and always will have the ability to heal ourselves. This knowledge is returning to us now, and knowledge is power. How we use this power ultimately will determine what happens to us. And while it seems as though many are denying their personal power, a more sustainable system of co-creation is emerging. We were never meant to simply survive or to give our power over to another. All of our "survival" needs are constantly and spontaneously being met, but when we are cut off from the source from which everything flows, we can't see that. It's like the parable of the blind men and the elephant. When our perception becomes limited, the universe meets our expectations of lack. We have been cut off largely due to our own fear, specifically fear of lack. In essence, we have cut the branch on which we are sitting. Self-heal reminds us that we are always being supported and we always have everything we need in order to heal.

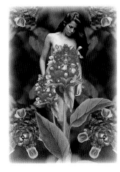

THE DEVA SPEAKS

What is this emotion that you call *love,* to which you aspire with no conditions? Humans have only ever known conditional love. Your conditions for love are based on survival. The elements have always been here to serve your evolution, and their love alone is unconditional on this plane.

It is a law in your dimension that there will always be this struggle toward the light of love, a struggle that will continue as long as you take form in a dimension of duality and separation. Your notion of unconditional love is actually a field of love emanating from a Central Sun that you have already begun to perceive. When the need to survive is no longer upon you, you will enter this vibrational field of love. No conditions as you presently know them exist in this field, for love *is* what is. In this field I have grown my medicine for you, and through this field we will walk together as I show you the way home to unconditional love.

Out of my great love for you, I have evolved my medicine for your body and for your soul. This creation was both conditional and intentional in order to manifest it in your physical reality. You had a need, the conditions were accessed and met, and then we developed the seed. This medicine has been essential to your survival. When you no longer need to survive in your present form and are ready to shift into your light body, you will find yourself immersed in that from which you came, the field of love, and we will become co-creators who play in yet other dimensional fields and planes of existence.

Honor your bodies. They are made up of the same elements as my own. This is how I *know* you. Should you in turn choose to know me, then focus on me, communicate with me, and take me into your body. This will create an intimacy that is the context and foundation for all healing and is my desire for you. Should you walk barefoot on the earth where I grow, I will read your signs carried to me by the elementals of the earth and learn of your imbalances. I will adjust my chemistry so that you can heal yourself with my medicine.

My condition for you has always been this: that you retrieve the lost fragments of your soul so that all of humanity can walk through the door I am holding open for you. It is not possible to walk into the light of a Central Sun while your souls are fragmented. You must gather and weave the pieces together so that your fabric is healed. You must self-heal and allow all that does not serve your evolution toward the light to be the dross that burns away. Know that what you hold most dear must eventually surrender to its own direction. Unconditional love is not something that you do or something that is contained within you; it is what you are made of and what contains you. It is a resonant field created by a Central Sun, where your soul is warmed and awakened.

I will tell you a story now of a quiet little village at the foot of a mountain by a river, where a child was born to a mother who had no father by her side to help raise the child. This child was well loved by the entire village, who took it upon themselves to help raise it. This was an extraordinary child, as it had no sexual organs and could not reproduce itself, and it had eyes that never focused on you the way a normal child's eyes would focus. And this child had no language that could be understood, yet all perfectly understood its communications. And while it had no language, it had a sweet laugh that tinkled and chimed like the village bells that called the people to gather, a laugh that reminded the villagers of the bells of the wandering goatherd.

It was not thought when this child was born that it would live, because there was something not quite right with its heart, and in fact the child did not live a very long life. When the day came that it chose to leave this life, it called all the villagers together with the tinkling of its laughter and without using a single word. And when all the villagers, who had loved this child for the whole of its life, stopped what they were doing and gathered together, they witnessed a most miraculous thing. As they waited and focused their attention on their beloved child, whom they had raised since birth, the child took in the whole of what was before it with unfocused eyes, and then the child simply dematerialized right in front of their eyes.

Where did it go? The villagers were shocked and amazed, and they speculated as to where it had gone and on what they had just gazed. Some said it was the work of evil, and some said it was a miracle. Some were angry, and some were relieved. No one was indifferent, and all were grief-stricken, and they all raised their hands to their hearts and felt something within them stir. A piece of them had gone home. A piece of them had returned. And with one whole heart, they turned to continue the work of their day, knowing that when it was their time to return home, they would be warmed by the fire of their labors and greeted by the sound of laughter and bells.

And so in your loving, without the condition of judgment, may you find your way home not only to unconditional love, but also home to yourself, where you love what you are and where you know that all that you are is connected within a field of love, a field from which you have come and to which you shall return. Your true mother carries within her the womb of all possibilities. She is your Mother Earth, the source of your sustenance and your renewal. Your true father is the spirit that carries the spark of creation, the light that lives within. When you are born to a mother who has no father by her side, you are missing a whole half of who you are. When you are born on Earth and trauma causes your spirit to flee, it seems as if you are condemned to search endlessly for this lost thing. But spirit also lives in the realm of the heavens and knows no earthly bounds.

I observe you not from a point of light, but from a grid that is multidimensional and contains your Earth and our star system, the Pleiades, which you call the Seven Sisters. This is why we are seven species within one genus, which is as you have identified us. From our perspective, Earth is part of the limitless heavens, where spirit lives and knows no bounds, and from your perspective, Earth is your three-dimensional mother, where you are bound by matter. When you collectively love all that you are, as the villagers loved their child, spirit will return. And spirit, which is the spark of life in all matter and able to spontaneously combust at will, will then become free of form and return to the field of love. It is the father in sacred union with the mother, the spark of life entering the womb of infinite possibilities that creates a New Earth. When the father returns, when spirit returns, then we know we are home. There is no need to seek to grow spiritually, for you are already spiritualized matter. Seek to grow in your emotional, physical, and mental bodies so that you may fully embody your spirit. Just as I grow toward the light, die, and return to the earth in my service to you, so will you grow toward the light of a Central Sun, die to your three-dimensional form, and take on a new light body in service to the entire universe.

For a long time now you have been on the spiral path of evolution, born over and over again. Each time you have gone in search of your father and then returned to the earth, only to begin the journey all over again at a higher octave. This time is different. In the field of unconditional love there are no polarities. You have fragmented your souls and peopled the earth with fragmented souls. And you have had enough experience doing this that you are now feeling the urge to move on, to move up the spiral ladder. It is indeed time to move on and to become the human being in love. When people love and care for one another, when you love yourself for the perfection of your imperfection and learn to be one with the heart-of-the-earth, spirit will fill the void and make whole what was previously torn apart. You are not weeds that need pruned and plucked and ethnically cleansed, but precious and beloved among species. This knowing, this power, this healing lives in your heart. I am the heart-of-the-earth. When I feel your love and you feel mine, then your gift to me becomes my gift of sustainable life to you. When love returns to the heart of the people, then each one of you will remember your soul's purpose. As each one of you grows in this purpose, just as I am growing toward the solar light, you will grow toward a Central Sun and become the healing that you seek. Each one of you has the power to heal yourself, to become whole and healed. Seek first to heal yourself, to self-heal, and I will guide you to the center of the Medicine Wheel Garden and a new level of consciousness, where you will become unconditional love.

Weeds

I learn more about God
From weeds than from roses;
Resilience springing
Through the smallest chink of hope
In the absolute of concrete.
Small seeds secreted
Under man's designings;
Roads and city plans,
The humourless utopias
Of arid dreams.
It seems God smiles:
A head of gold
So delicate yet strength enough
To bring temples to their knees
In time.
What is left of Greece
Is the work of weeds:
A humble persistence
Of unobserved beauty
The force of life enduring
The follies of men.

PHILLIP PULFREY

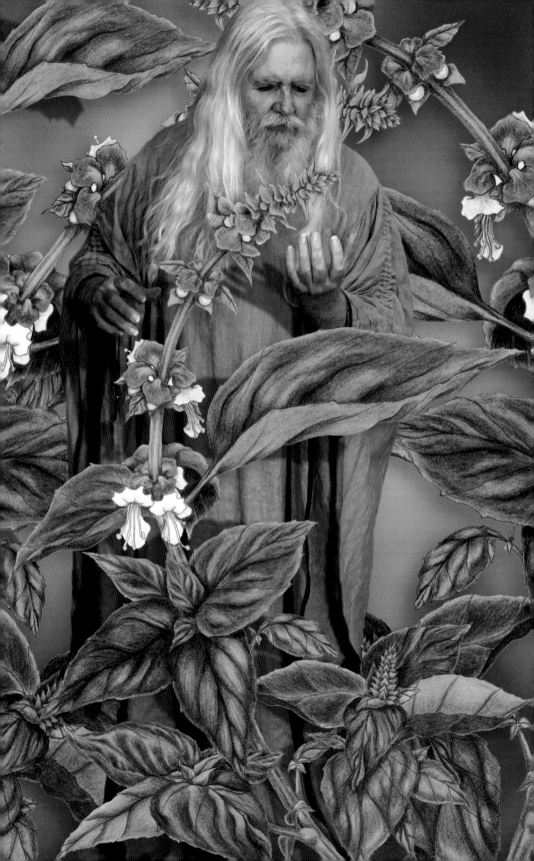

Sweet Basil

Ocimum basilicum

Sovereignty

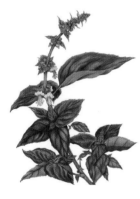

Ocimum basilicum, the sweet-smelling basil that is the king of the herbs, presents with square, branching stems; opposite leaves; and tiny black seeds. The flowers are small and arranged in a terminal spike; flower color and leaf size, shape, and texture vary by species. Decorative and delicious, sweet basil is a tender, low-growing herb that resides in both the tropical and subtropical regions of the Old and New Worlds.

Sweet basil, like so many of the aromatic herbs, is a member of the easily and widely cultivated Lamiaceae family of mints. You have only to crush it between your fingers to release the essence of its scent. The genus name, *Ocimum,* meaning "smell," alludes to the sweet and aromatic odor of these plants.

Basilicum, which stems from the ancient Greek *basileus,* meaning "sovereign" or "king," is a word that has been passed down through antiquity. A related word is *basilica,* an architectural style that first appeared as the center of public power in ancient Rome and Greece, whose halls of business

165

and trade evolved into courts of law. Sometimes basilicas were constructed at pagan temple sites, and they have even been compared to ancient Egyptian halls.*

Jesus and innumerable martyrs were condemned to death in basilicas, and they were later venerated in them, after basilicas received religious acceptance as places of worship. The proper names Basil, Basileus, and the feminine Basilissa were given to martyrs, saints, and kings. In yet another form of the word, *basilicus,* meaning "dragon," we find the root for *basilisk,* the mythological king of the serpents that could kill you with its eyes. Some believed that sweet basil oil was an antidote to the basilisk's venom, and it is still used to treat the venom of scorpion stings.

Sweet basil is considered to have originated in India and Persia prior to being brought to Greece by Alexander the Great. During the Hellenistic period, which followed the conquest of Alexander the Great and began with his death in 323 BCE, a great deal of Egyptian and Middle Eastern culture was brought into Greek civilization. Sweet basil is thought to have been a part of this cultural exchange, making its way across Asia and Africa to Europe, where it acquired the Latin root of its name. If you were to travel throughout the region surrounding the Mediterranean Sea, you would find sweet basil growing extensively. In the late 1600s the colonists brought sweet basil to America, where it is still highly prized for its culinary and medicinal value.

The true botanical identity of sweet basil is questionable and of some scientific concern, because it has a tendency to be promiscuous and cross-pollinate. This has resulted in a large number of subspecies. Sweet basil is the most familiar, but the list of basil species and cultivars is extensive and exotic. The world of *Ocimum basilicum* brings us cultivars like 'Cinnamon,' 'Thai,' 'Genovese,' 'Persian,' 'Spicy Globe,' and 'Dark Opal,' to name a few. 'Lemon Basil' and 'Lime Basil' are *Ocimum americanum* cultivars. Another important species is holy basil, *Ocimum sanctum,* known in India as *tulsi,* where it is venerated by Hindus and a principal plant in Ayurvedic medicine. Tulsi is believed to be the "elixir of life" and thought to promote longevity.

---

*Roman architect Vitruvius discussed basilicas in *De Architectura,* a treatise on architecture probably written around 25 BCE and the only contemporary source on classical architecture to have survived in its entirety.

Sweet basil's many herbal uses include culinary, landscaping, medicinal, and spiritual, and the essential oil can be found in fragrances and insect repellents. Cultivated largely as a culinary herb and often associated with Italian cuisine, basil is excellent in tomato-based dishes. It is also used cooked or raw in sauces, stews, salad dressings, vegetable and meat dishes, bean dishes, vinegars, confectionery products, and the liqueur Chartreuse. While sweet basil can be successfully dried, it is best used fresh in cooking, as the dried herb loses most of its flavor. The fresh herb smells of clove and tastes somewhat like anise. As the main ingredient in the original pesto, *pesto alla genovese*, a sauce originating in northern Italy, sweet basil is crushed along with garlic and combined with olive oil, coarse salt, and grated hard cheese. Now a popular dish throughout Europe and North America, pesto has evolved to include the addition of minced pine nuts or walnuts. While pesto is commonly used on pasta, it has also been traditionally added to potatoes and green beans. Basil is also an important spice in Thai, Laotian, and Vietnamese cooking. When added to food, it is warming and carminative, aiding in digestion. Sweet basil is an excellent source of vitamin K; a very good source of vitamin A, calcium, and iron; and a good source of vitamin C, magnesium, potassium, and manganese. It is best not overcooked.

As a landscaping herb, sweet basil is an annual whose flowers attract bees in the summer. After insect pollination, the petals fall off and what appear to be four round seeds develop inside the bilabiate calyx, or sepals. These round "seeds" are actually dry fruits called achenes that contain a single seed. Unlike most mints, sweet basil has four stamens and a pistil. These are not pushed under the upper lip of the petals, but lie over the top. It grows to approximately two feet in height, requires full sun and a light to sandy, well-drained soil, and should be planted in late spring and harvested in early fall. Companion planting sweet basil next to tomatoes can help ward off the white fly that plagues them. Sweet basil's essential oil also acts as a larvicide against houseflies and mosquitoes, and the potted plant was frequently placed on windowsills and near doorways to keep the flies out.

Traditionally sweet basil has been used to treat a vast array of ailments, from headaches and nausea to sinus congestion and fevers. Energetically sweet basil is both warming and calming, and as a tea, it stimulates the lungs, calms the stomach, and dries internal dampness. It is widely used in aromatherapy due to its volatile oil. The steamed, distilled essential oil of sweet basil contains high amounts of camphor compounds, known to possess antibacterial and antifungal properties and useful against some strains of *Staphylococcus* and *Candida*.

A soap made from sweet basil essential oil not only smells pleasant, but also works well as an antibacterial soap and may be effective in treating acne. Sweet basil, like oregano, has been shown to have antioxidant activity, as well as antispasmodic and anti-inflammatory properties, and may prove useful in treating inflammatory bowel disease and arthritis. Beta-caryophyllene (BCP) is the constituent in sweet basil's essential oil that blocks chemical signals that lead to inflammation.* This constituent is the same one found in cloves and in *Cannabis sativa,* only sweet basil does the job without triggering the *Cannabis* plant's mood-altering effects.

The many rituals, beliefs, legends, and lore surrounding sweet basil have for centuries brought forth a mix of symbolism that includes the polar opposites of love and fear, danger and protection, life and death. But its strongest symbolism may be that of offering protection while invoking inner strength. To the Cherokee it is a "West Medicine" that focuses on the internal aspects of the physical body. Sweet basil is one of many herbs used by the Egyptians for embalming. They believed it opened the gates to the next world as a person was leaving the physical body. The Egyptians also gathered sweet basil at midday and dried it during the astrological sign of Scorpio. It was then ground into a powder and burned in equal parts with myrrh to symbolize the divine union of god and goddess. As a witch's herb it is believed to have magical powers and is used in spells to attract money and love, and to repel evil.

One legend tells us that fresh basil placed in the left hand of a lover will tell that person's true intentions. If the king of the herbs stays fresh while being held in the left hand, then our lover will stay devoted, and if it withers, then our lover will quickly leave us. A pagan ritual later co-opted by Christians in the Ukraine is that of the *didukh,* which literally means "grand-

---

*Beta-caryophyllene is shown to selectively bind to the cannabinoid receptor type-2 and exert significant anti-inflammatory effects.[1]

father spirit."[2] The didukh is a ceremonial sheaf made from the best stalks of grain gathered during the fall harvest and decorated with flowers, ribbons, and a small wreath of sweet basil and other herbs. It is ritualistically carried into the home at Christmastime or on the winter solstice, and it is believed to house the spirits of family members passed on and those yet to be born. When the holiday season comes to its close, the didukh is carried out of the home and scattered across the fields with prayers for continuance.

THE DIVINATION

When you enter the Medicine Wheel Garden, enter with reverence, for the king of the herbs awaits you. If sweet basil has called you to his side in the garden, breathe deeply of his royal scent and know that you *are* love. Within each one of us is the polarity of the sacred feminine and divine masculine. When these two marry, we achieve sovereignty. It is a marriage of the soul, reuniting us with our divine purpose. We come from the One and return to the One. We are one with all things—one spirit, one mind. Only the human ego knows separation from the sacred and the divine. The integration of the opposites inside of us, light and dark, masculine and feminine, right brain and left brain, is what brings us into wholeness. It is from this place of an integrated whole that great leaders are born. All the leaders, saints, and prophets whom we hold in high esteem know this principle of oneness. It is through the field of love that we unite, love of self and of others. This is what our greatest teachers have tried to teach us. "If thine eye be single, thy whole body shall be full of light" (Matthew 6:22).

Sweet basil asks us to enter the interior, to look inside of ourselves for the answers and for guidance. Our body is the house of law, the temple, the basilica. The laws of nature are not the laws of man. We have become so afraid that even our local governments can no longer manage us, and we have begun to look to an even larger global government to manage our world. We pass more and more laws in an effort to manage and control the masses. But no amount of external management will quell the search for sovereignty of our true self. If we can start by recognizing the beauty in the exterior world of manifestation—in the marriage of mother earth and father sky, yin and yang, sun and moon, heaven and earth—then we can begin to recognize our own internal beauty, for each world is a mirror of the other.

Not vacillating between dualities but flowing between polarities is where we find the mystical experience of alchemy that is part of the "as above, so below" mysteries. We may visualize this flowing between polarities as energy moving in the pattern of a figure eight. A myriad of archetypes dance before us, showing us the way to sacred union: Shakti and Shiva, Venus and Mars, Isis and Osiris. All are unique expressions of the One, and it is through the integration of the dimension of duality that our perception shifts and we experience the divine union of opposites.

Shifting our perception from rational reductionism to a more holistic perspective brings us into alignment with the natural world and the principles of life-force energy. Cruelty and inhumanity are the result of linear thinking and an old story in our human history. Linear thinking, which is left-brain driven, doesn't take into consideration the subtle yet profound consequences of decisions based on perceived survival needs. Nor does it feel into these consequences, further severing the creative and intuitive part of us, perpetuating an ongoing cycle of soul loss and diminishing spirit. Nature's wisdom is that of constant flux between stillness and receptivity, activity and forceful energy. In a culture that values one and undervalues the other, as is the case in our fast-paced, activity-driven society, which doesn't take the time to reflect and meditate, these imbalances play out in perversions of the natural flow.

Forceful energy is necessary, but it has become confused with aggression. There is no need to defend anything aggressively when standing in one's personal power. Protection is automatically afforded to the sovereign. A single masculine deity and male domination arises from predominantly left-brain thinking. Along with this domination comes a long history of defensive and offensive violence. The opposite is true in right-brain thinking, such as can be seen in Native America, where the supreme being is expressed in the feminine archetypes of White Buffalo Calf Woman (Dakota), Deer Mother (Taos), Corn Mother (Hopi), and Changing Woman (Navajo). For the Native American, the woman and mother comes first.

It is time to regain and reclaim the fullness of our human potential using the whole of our brain and a new understanding of what it means to be whole.

Perhaps we can now begin to see sweet basil's association with the polarity of fear and death as two sides of the same coin, the unconscious shadow side that requires an antidote to the venom. "But if thine eye be evil, thy whole body shall be full of darkness" (Matthew 6:23). Sacred marriage is the antidote. Honoring the light *and* dark forces within us results in a whole new mind, one in which we integrate the rational with the intuitive and become the visionaries and leaders that inspire a higher octave of humanity.

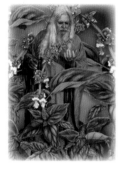

THE DEVA SPEAKS

I have been here since before the fires of your own hell destroyed your memory of me. I am the Sovereign King. It is my essence that is returning to you now, for what good is it to recover the sacred feminine if there is no divine masculine with whom to marry? I reflect what is in your gene pool, for I am polyamorous. I have become many species in one. This mixing of your blood is for a reason, so that you may know yourselves as part of a larger whole. My evolution is in service to the highest good. As you expand, I expand.

The Dragon King is born again and again with a sword in his hand and a sense of entitlement. Driven either to prove himself worthy of treasure he believes is rightfully his or to be coddled and spoiled and paralyzed by fear, he awaits the silver cup and spoon. The treasure that you seek and your source of abundant flow are the domain of the sacred feminine. What you call a "sensitive new-age man," is the new masculine returning in the form of the Sweet King. He is struggling to reclaim his lost feminine part, the other half of himself. The queen must come down off her throne and stand eye to eye with her own inner tyrant so that she may come to terms with masculine abandonment and call the king back to her, for he is the other half of who she is.

Raise your sword of light, my dear Sweet King, for it is charged with the power of a million suns. Take this power into your body as I take it into my own. Let it shine through your lingam, as your sexual and spiritual body becomes one body. Let its light penetrate your queen as together you create a new heaven and a New Earth. As you reconcile your now separate but soon to be united bodies, you become sovereign unto yourself. This magnetic completion repels what does not serve and attracts your heart's true desire.

Your going-away-from time is your returning-to-now time. In the space of your light body, time is measured differently. Pure presence flows from the door of creativity I hold open for you. My evolution into light body is the result of a divine marriage of opposites, which is serving your journey now. Behold my glorious flower stalk! Look into my eyes and know thyself. Smell the richness of my royal scent and know yourself once again as the sovereign being that you are. You carry this same essence in your own bodies. You have named it pheromones. Dear human ones, made of the same water, earth, and light as my own body, breathe deeply of this essence activated through your sexual union and be transported into dimensions that await your return. You were meant to ascend. It is written in your codes. Awaken the divine masculine. Marry it with the sacred feminine, and know the sweetness of sacred union. I am open to the source of divine essence.

The time of the tyrant rule of your patriarchy is ending. This is not a time of returning to matriarchal rule, but a time of integration. You are complete unto yourself and will learn to trust your own inner authority and guidance. The reason you have been so easy to control is because you did not want to be in charge of yourself. You were the only one who was ever in need of self-rule. There is no escape from power or its lessons. When you become a sovereign being, you will cease to source outside yourself and erase the belief that you are powerless. The external sourcing, the plundering and pillaging came from an ignorance of this sovereign self. You were yet a young species who chose to explore these polarities of yourself.

What was once in shadow comes to the surface as it dies. In the Age of Pisces, which is presently ending, your love turned into dependency, your compassion into pity, your forgiveness into defensiveness, and your spirituality into religion. But the time has come for you to mature into compassionate, loving, and spiritual beings and release your attachment to the outcome. In the coming age of the Aquarian shaman and king, the old king will die and the new archetypes of truth, multidimensionality, spiritual freedom, and creativity will be born. It is time to come home. Be at peace with this earth. Let the sweetness of this knowing command your hands as leaders, visionaries, and teachers. It has always been so.

The Song of Sweet Basil

Basil, Sweet Basil, the love of my life
You have given me pause from the struggle and
        strife
Strong in your gifts
You embody the light
Calm in your healing
You embody the shift
A leader of men whole unto themselves
Sweet Basil you are singing us, bringing us
        home
The bard of the garden is calling us home
Calling us home, ever home to ourselves

THEA SUMMER DEER

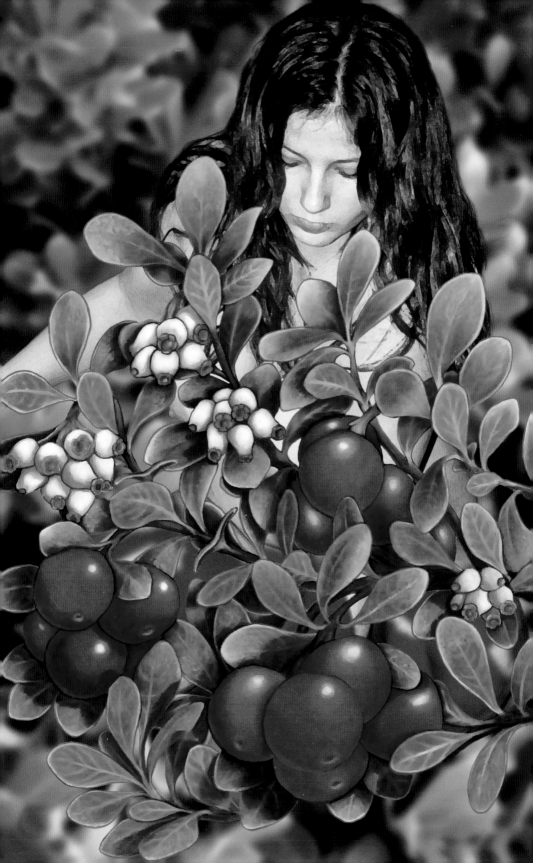

Uva Ursi

Arctostaphylos uva ursi

Introspection

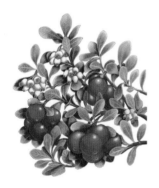

The bright red berry of *Arctostaphylos uva ursi*, or bearberry, is one of the few foods for bear and other wildlife available in the winter. Both the genus and species names refer to bears and grapes: *uva* means "grape" and *ursi* means "bear." *Arctostaphylos* combines the Greek word for bear, *arkto*, with the word for grape, *staphyle*. While black bear and grizzly bear eat uva ursi berries in the autumn, it is especially important to them in the early spring when coming out of hibernation.

However, it is the small, leathery, and ovate leaf of uva ursi that is used medicinally. *Arctostaphylos* is a member of the heath, or Ericaceae, family, which also includes manzanita, a common shrub of the chaparral biome of western North America. Unlike manzanita, uva ursi is found in a much wider range of habitats, including the arctic, coastal, and mountainous regions of North America, Asia, and Europe. It is a ground-hugging, evergreen, perennial sub-shrub with long stems that often appear interwoven. Those stems form a compact and intricate mat that offers ground cover to small animals

175

and birds. The deep roots of uva ursi prevent erosion from the nutrient-poor soils and steep, dry, sunny slopes where it often grows.

The best way to propagate uva ursi is by obtaining stem cuttings in the fall. They must be protected during their first winter, as they take up to a year to root. They are difficult to start from seed, and seedling growth is slow for the first three years.

Uva ursi thrives in acidic soils and is totally dependent on a symbiotic relationship with a fungus, an arbutoid mycorrhiza that grows in and around its roots to provide nutrients not readily available in the poor soils where it is typically found. Like all members of the Ericaceae family, its flowers contain both male and female parts. Pale pink, drooping, bell-shaped clusters bloom in the summer and are primarily wind pollinated. The plant produces a bright red berry in the fall containing four to five seeds, and the berries remain on the plant throughout the winter. Foraging animals and gravity disperse the seeds. These slow-germinating seeds have hard coats and may remain dormant in the finer layers of topsoil for long periods of time, undamaged by drought or fire.

Another common name for uva ursi is kinnikinnick, an Algonquian word meaning "mixture." Most likely this refers to the tradition of mixing the leaves with other herbs and tobacco. This mixture may be used as a tobacco substitute and is a popular remedy to help people quit smoking. Tobacco is gradually weaned out of the mixture, which minimizes the withdrawal symptoms, while the mixture itself satisfies the need for an oral fixation. Once the tobacco is gone from the mixture, one can reduce the frequency of use. Used during ceremonies or in tribal councils, kinnikinnick was thought to calm and clear the mind, as well as to help bring visions and guidance. American Indians also made an ash-colored dye from the leaves and fruit, dried the berries for use in rattles or as beads, and used the plant's tannic acid to preserve leather. Bearberries were considered a survival food and were added to winter stews and pounded into pemmican, a concentrated mixture of fat and protein that can be stored long term and was invented by the native peoples of North America.

Although bears eat the uva ursi berries, their nutritional quality and energy value is actually very low, but because of this they spoil very slowly.

The plant's popularity is probably due only to the fact that it can be found in the deep of winter when other food sources are unavailable. Elk, bighorn sheep, mountain goat, deer, moose, and other wildlife eat the berries from fall into spring and also graze on the vegetation, but domestic livestock avoid it. Despite its low nutritional value, it is possible that uva ursi has some medicinal value for these wild animals, though this has yet to be documented.

Uva ursi has been used medicinally since at least the second century by the early Romans. There is evidence of its use by Native Americans as a remedy for urinary tract infections. Before the discovery of sulfa drugs and antibiotics, an infusion of uva ursi leaves was a common treatment for bladder infections and inflammation (cystitis), and it is still used for this purpose. The astringent action of tannins also helps to shrink and tighten mucous membranes and reduce inflammation. An oil infusion of the leaves can be made into a salve and used for skin sores and cradle cap. Green leaves should be selectively harvested for quality early in the autumn and gently dried.

Scientific research has discovered that uva ursi's infection-fighting properties are due to the chemical compound arbutin,* which exerts antibacterial activity in the urinary tract as it is excreted. Arbutin in uva ursi leaves, which is hydrolyzed by intestinal bacteria and skin microflora into hydroquinone, inhibits melanin production, which prevents the skin from making the pigment responsible for skin color. Both arbutin and hydroquinone have powerful antioxidant abilities and when applied to the skin can provide photo-protection against damage caused by free radicals. Paradoxically this is also the role of melanin, which hydroquinone inhibits.

While arbutin is a naturally occurring substance that research claims may reduce cancer risk, hydroquinone on the other hand can cause liver damage and increases cancer risk, specifically bladder cancer. Furthermore, emerging research has made a clear association between deficiencies in exposure to sunlight (necessary for melanin formation) and bladder cancer, with the highest incidence of bladder cancer occurring among white males living in the Northern Hemisphere.[1]

---

*Arbutin is both an ether and a glycoside and is technically known as hydroquinone-beta-D-glucoside.

Hydroquinone is the primary topical ingredient for inhibiting melanin production in popular skin-whitening creams, pills, soaps, and lotions. Skin lightening is a controversial subject, not only as it relates to the detrimental effects on health from reduced UV protection and toxicity, but also with regard to issues of identity, self-image, and race. Skin-whitening creams are used extensively in India, and they are marketed to a wide variety of groups, from rural villagers to urban professionals, throughout Asia, Africa, Latin America, and the Middle East. Arbutin was very popular in Japan at one time for its skin-lightening properties. However, geisha now paint their skin white rather than bleaching it for ceremonies that celebrate their culture and background.

The whitening cream industry is estimated to be worth around $432 million in India and $7 billion in China. Due to the increasing trend of targeting male consumers and promoting endorsements by celebrities, such as Indian actor Shahrukh Khan, sales have increased significantly in non-European markets in recent years.[2] Additionally it is used for genital and anal whitening, in an attempt to reduce the darker pigmentation of the genital and perianal area. Hydroquinone has been shown to cause leukemia in mice and other animals, and the European Union banned it from cosmetics in 2001. But it keeps showing up in bootleg creams in the developing world and is sold in the United States as an over-the-counter drug.

While arbutin is a natural product derived from the leaves of uva ursi and an alternative to synthetically produced hydroquinone, the issue remains that separating the active ingredient of a plant from the whole of its constituents, especially for reasons of manipulating our bodies to conform to a projected image of beauty, has far-reaching consequences. The perception of beauty as being something removed from nature has been the subject of much artistic expression and debate. We are incredibly creative beings who continuously make and remake ourselves and the world around us. The inspiration and intention behind our creations beg to come into consciousness so that we may rebuild ourselves more in harmony with the beauty of the natural world. Beauty is a matter of perception, and learning how to walk in beauty begins when we look within.

THE DIVINATION

A mirror resides in the west of the Medicine Wheel Garden, and it is made of reflective sheets of falling rain and standing pools of water. Look deep into water, for it is a reflection of your deepest self. It is also a gift from the elementals, charged with the power of love, which brings life to the plants and ultimately to all of us.

Uva ursi's Bear Medicine is not only reflected in the power animal for which it is named, but also in the deep reservoir of the kidneys and urinary tract system. Behind the Medicine Wheel Garden dwells the Medicine Bear Lodge. It is a place of deep introspection during the winter months, when animals hibernate and all of nature slows or comes to a standstill. The shadow cave, or the darkness of the void, is where we learn about the creation of form from the formless. It is where we enter the dreamtime. Within this watery world of the urinary tract system and the kidneys, which are the deepest and most protected organs in the body, we see uva ursi's affect on health and well-being. From the darkness of the void, up through the watery depths of our unconscious emotions, we are dreamed into form and given consciousness. The feminine mysteries represented by water, emotion, darkness, and intuition speak of this metaphorically. It is from the dark womb of the Great Mother that we take our watery birth.

The next step in our evolution will be to learn how to enter the void, where we will discover that all form comes from the same source. The importance of caring for oneself at the deepest level by nourishing the kidneys is something that has been understood in Chinese medicine for thousands of years. The kidneys in the energetic model of Chinese medicine are seen as the repository of fear. Fear is what causes us to seek to control and to be controlled. If we are to be free of the limitation of fear, we must heal at the deepest levels of our being. Introspection allows us to surrender our need to control what is happening outside of ourselves. When we no longer fear what is in the shadow cave, we will be free of the projection of fear. In truth, shadow and light cannot exist without each other in this dimension of duality. The opportunity that we are being given is to embrace the shadow and no longer project our fear onto others. As we integrate our shadow, we step into the light of a greater understanding of our humanity.

While uva ursi's medicine may help to heal a urinary tract infection, it is important to use it energetically by journeying inward with the spirit of this plant as an ally. Within the cave of our inner knowing is the answer to the question of how to take better care of our health. Then we would never need uva ursi's physical medicine. When we enter the inner cave of our being, the seat of our consciousness, fear can no longer take residence in our physical body, and we will have learned how to nurture ourselves at the deepest level. And when we take the time to honor the season of our evolution by entering the silence, then we can begin to realize that we are all unique expressions emanating from the same source. At this level of self-realization, there is no need to control or manipulate out of fear or lack.

We are currently being challenged in so many ways to find alternative solutions to the human condition, and if we honor the call to look within, we will emerge reborn in the spring, full of glorious new beginnings. How can we create the vision of a New Earth if we do not first seek a vision? We call forth the silence by calming the mind and heeding the rhythm of the seasons. Introspection is presently needed. When we call on the spirit medicine of uva ursi, a great ally will be made available to assist us on the inner journey. Whether you keep the leaves and berries in a potpourri by your bedside, sip it gingerly in a leaf tea from time to time, smoke it in your peace pipe, or use it as a smudge, uva ursi will tend to your need for silence and introspection.

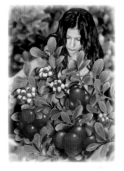

THE DEVA SPEAKS

I stand before you as a living testament to the necessity of healthy interdependent relationships. I coexist with those who assist in feeding me when no other sustenance can be found. In turn I feed those who can find no other sustenance. I have evolved simultaneously with the invisible ones you call fungus. My evolution has unfolded simultaneously with the four-leggeds and the winged ones who eat of me, and with you, my beloved two-leggeds. I have loved you for so long, providing berries for your stews and smoke for your prayers. I have helped to keep the forest canopy over your head and the earth held firm beneath my roots, when it might have otherwise washed away. We are not separate, and if we did not feed each other in our time of need, we would not be here to share our dance among the stars on this most beautiful of water planets. As deeply as your imagination has pursued the reaches of outer space, so must you now look within yourselves to find the depth of who you really are, why you are here, and where you have come from.

When you follow the path of the bear and enter the silence of the cave, you will cross a certain threshold. Many mystics before you have known the power of this place that is being made readily available to all of human consciousness through tools such as my medicine. Native peoples across the whole of your beloved planet have practiced a purification ritual for millennia for the purpose of entering the darkness and making contact with the void. While these rituals and ceremonies are valuable tools that have served your evolution, the time of practicing is coming to an end and the time of living this reality is at hand. You no longer need to seek tools that exist outside of yourself. The most powerful of tools for turning the evolutionary key live right inside of you, and you were given access to them when you took your first breath. Learn to journey through the power of your breath to the inner cave of higher knowing. When you cross this threshold you will enter a new era, for you will then hold the knowledge of the void, where all form takes its birth. And you will dream your dreams and own them, for the time of living the separate dream of another has ended. I am a window to your soul.

In the deep snows of winter, when the bears are asleep, the bark of trees and my berries see the wildlife that lives in the cold lands of the north through the long nights of winter white. And in the spring, when the wise one wakes from her slumber, her belly full of promise, I feed her. The same is true for you. It was necessary for you to first enter the darkness of her cave and to fall asleep, gestating the promise of what will be born through you when you emerge into the light. I will feed your soul when you emerge, for I am a light being who has taken form to assist you in this return to the light. The northern lights are already speaking to you as the earth goes through her changes.

Indeed, the light is shifting, and what is changing inside you is the evolution of consciousness.

Look within yourself. There you will find the truth of interdependence and inner connectedness. There is no difference between you and other human beings; they are your family and share your same Earth. You all walk on two legs, breathe the same air, and are always touching through your Mother Earth. Supremacy is an illusion, an attempt to rise above what you believe to be common and mundane. The belief that a supreme being exists somewhere outside of yourself is a projection. You are a supreme being. While I, too, belong to a family of many different sizes, shapes, and colors, we are all of the same Earth, living under one sky, fed by the same water. The same sun influences the color of my body and the color of your skin. Do not seek to alter that which has been given to you in total perfection. While you may have examined my fruits and found them to be of little value, this is exactly the medicine needed at this time. Trust that everything has a divine purpose. Even when life seems futile and you begin to sink into the long, hard winter of despair, be aware that there is fruit that will outlast the famine. This is my gift to you, and it lives in your soul.

My medicine is for your soul to know its true home and holds the power to awaken the light within you. While you are presently in body, the time is coming when you will return to light. Practice looking inside of yourself to discover this light. Through introspection you will know the truth of who you really are. We are all interconnected, and together we will lift each other up to the light of a New Earth.

Winter

I love these winter skies
and the ice that hangs from eaves.
The view through barren trees
reveals what could not before be seen.

In winter cardinals dressed in red
dance upon a stage of white,
and a brilliant star of dazzling light
guides me west, and home at night.

I love these mountain woods,
where the bobcat watches as I stand
before the fire to warm my hands.
We welcome winter solstice with its breath of
     cold demand.

In winter the black bear sleeps
where I may join her in my dreams.
She takes me down by inner streams
and reveals what could not before be seen.

THEA SUMMER DEER

Herbal Actions

Herbal actions are the specific effects that an herb may have on the human body. The terms describe the symptoms that herbs can help mediate. Below are herbal actions for the herbs discussed in this book. The herbs that contain these healing attributes are listed in parentheses.

Alterative: Gradually restores proper function to the body, increasing overall health and vitality (red clover, self-heal).

Anticatarrhal: Removes excess mucus and is mainly used for ear, nose, and throat infections (sagebrush, uva ursi).

Antidepressant: *See* nervine.

Antifungal: Kills or inhibits fungal growth (calendula, sweet basil).

Anti-inflammatory: Soothes inflammations or reduces inflammatory response (borage, calendula, comfrey, sacred datura, lavender, self-heal, sweet basil).

Antimicrobial: Destroys or resists pathogenic microorganisms (calendula, lavender, lemon balm, rosemary, self-heal, sagebrush, uva ursi).

Antispasmodic: Eases muscle cramps and alleviates muscular tension. *See* nervine.

Antiviral: Interferes with specific steps in the viral replication process (lemon balm, self-heal).

Astringent: Shrinks tissues and reduces secretions, reduces irritation and is related to the presence of tannins (calendula, comfrey, rosemary, sagebrush, self-heal, uva ursi).

Bitter: Stimulates the flow of digestive juices (calendula, sagebrush, self-heal).

Carminative: Warms the digestive system and promotes healthy digestive system function (lavender, lemon balm, rosemary, self-heal, sweet basil).

Cholagogue: Stimulates the flow of bile from the liver (calendula, lemon balm, rosemary).

Demulcent: Soothes and protects irritated or inflamed tissue (borage, comfrey, uva ursi).

Diaphoretic: Promotes perspiration, helping to reduce fever and eliminate waste (borage, lemon balm).

Diuretic: Increases the production and elimination of urine (self-heal, uva ursi).

Emmenogogue: Stimulates menstrual flow and function (calendula, lavender, rosemary).

Expectorant: Stimulates the removal of mucus from the lungs as a relaxant or stimulant (red clover, comfrey, sagebrush).

Galactogogue: Stimulates lactation (borage).

Hepatic: Supporting to the liver (lemon balm).

Lymphatic: Stimulates lymphatic drainage (calendula).

Nervine: Acts on the nervous system as a tonic, relaxant, or stimulant. Includes hypnotics, analgesics, antispasmodics, antidepressants, and adaptogens (borage, calendula, lavender, lemon balm, red clover, rosemary, self-heal, sweet basil).

Rubefacient: Stimulates a localized increase in blood flow (lavender, rosemary, sagebrush).

Tonic: Nurtures and strengthens the body (borage, calendula, lemon balm, self-heal).

Vulnerary: Promotes wound healing, primarily to heal the skin and may be used to heal internal wounds such as stomach ulcers (calendula, comfrey, self-heal).

Resources

BOOKS AND EDUCATIONAL MATERIALS

Michael C. Hirschi, F. William Simmons, Doug Peterson, and Ed Giles, *50 Ways Farmers Can Protect Their Groundwater*. Urbana-Champaign, Ill.: University of Illinois, Cooperative Extension Service, 1994.

Patricia Kyritsi Howell, *Basic Concepts of Energetic Herbalism*. A two-CD set available from BotanoLogos School for Herbal Studies. www.wildhealingherbs.com/bot_products.php

Michael Moore, founder of the Southwest School of Botanical Medicine. Extensive library of images, manuals, folios, lectures, and articles. www.swsbm.com/HOMEPAGE/HomePage.html

Susun Weed, *Herbal Medicine and Spirit Healing the Wise Woman Way*. Over 4,000 pages of complementary integrative health resources for women and men. www.susunweed.com

David Winston, RH (AHG), *Herbal Therapeutics*. Books, recordings, research, and articles. www.herbaltherapeutics.net

FIELD GUIDES

Steven Foster and James A. Duke, *Peterson's Field Guide to Medicinal Plants and Herbs*. New York: Houghton Mifflin Company, 2000.

Lawrence Newcomb, *Newcomb's Wildflower Guide*. New York: Little, Brown and Company, 1989.

ORGANIZATIONS AND ASSOCIATIONS

American Herbalists Guild, a nonprofit, educational organization that represents the goals and voices of herbalists specializing in the medicinal use of plants.
P.O. Box 230741, Boston, Massachusetts 02123
www.americanherbalistsguild.com

ATTRA is a project of the National Sustainable Agriculture Information Service, maintained by the National Center for Appropriate Technology.
http://attra.ncat.org

The Herb Society of America provides herbal profiles and guides.
9019 Kirtland Chardon Rd., Kirtland, Ohio 44094
www.herbsociety.org/herbs/profiles-and-guides.html

Less Lawn, creating sustainable landscapes.
www.lesslawn.com

National Herbalists Association of Australia is the publisher of the quarterly *Australian Journal of Medical Herbalism*.
PO Box 45, Concord West, NSW 2138 Australia
www.nhaa.org.au

SageSTEP (Sagebrush Steppe Treatment Evaluation Project) is a regional experiment to evaluate methods of sagebrush steppe restoration in the Great Basin.
www.sagestep.org/index.htm

United Plant Savers, an organization dedicated to preserving medicinal plants.
P.O. Box 400, East Barre, Vermont 05649
www.unitedplantsavers.org

Venus Rising Institute for the Shamanic Healing Arts
http://shamanicbreathwork.org

Frank Waters Foundation: Nurturing the Creative Spirit
www.frankwaters.org

WildEarth Guardians' Sagebrush Sea Campaign
www.sagebrushsea.org

TEACHERS AND PRACTITIONERS

Laura Cerwinske, teacher of transformational healing. She believes creativity
to be the supreme expression of power.
http://lauracerwinske.com

Eliot Cowan, author of *Plant Spirit Medicine* and founder of Blue Deer
Center. He teaches in the Huichol shamanic tradition.
www.bluedeer.org/teachers/eliot-cowan

Find an Herbalist: American Herbalist Guild provides a free brochure
of members who have received professional status and the title registered
herbalist, AHG.
www.americanherbalistsguild.com/fundamentals

Rosemary Gladstar, a pioneer in the herbal movement and author of
numerous books. She teaches extensively throughout the United States
and worldwide.
www.sagemt.com/rosemary-gladstar.html

Patricia Kyristi Howell, RH (AHG), founder and director of the
BotanoLogos School for Herbal Studies. She specializes in teaching about
Southern Appalachian medicinal herbs.
www.wildhealingherbs.com

Susun Weed, herbalist and author of women's health books. She is the
founder of Wise Woman University.
www.susunweed.com
www.wisewomanuniversity.org

David Winston, RH (AHG), is an herbalist and ethnobotanist with almost forty years of training in Cherokee, Chinese, and Western herbal traditions.
www.herbaltherapeutics.net

HERBAL SUPPLIERS

Hitchin Lavender, Cadwell Farm, Ickleford, Hitchin, Herts, SG5 3UA United Kingdom
www.hitchinlavender.com

Mountain Rose Herbs, Eugene, Oregon, offers quality organic herbal products and supports sustainable agriculture. Learn more about herbal education and find a list of herbal schools on their website.
www.mountainroseherbs.com

Native American Botanics, "Native American Herbs by Native Americans," is operated on the Pascua Yaqui reservation, southwest of Tucson, Arizona
www.nativeamericanbotanics.com

Notes

CALENDULA

1. William Shakespeare, *The Winter's Tale* (Whitefish, Mont.: Kessinger Publishing, 2010), act 4, scene 4.

COMFREY

1. Joseph M. Betz, Robert M. Eppley, Wendell C. Taylor, and D. Andrzejewski, "Determination of Pyrrolizidine Alkaloids in Commercial Comfrey Products," *Journal of Pharmaceutical Sciences* 83 (1994): 649–53.
2. Jane Brody, "Americans Gamble on Herbs as Medicine," *New York Times,* February 9, 1997.

SACRED DATURA

1. A. Avery, G. Amos, S. Satina, and J. Rietsema, *Blakeslee: The Genus Datura* (New York: Ronald Press, 1959), 4.
2. H. K. Bakhru, *Herbs That Heal: Natural Remedies for Good Health* (New Delhi, India: Orient Paperbacks, 1990), 81.
3. Paul J. Jackson, W. L. Anderson, J. G. DeWitt, H. Y. D. Ke, C. R. Kuske, R. M. Moncrief, and G. D. Rayson, "Accumulation of Toxic Metal Ions on Cell Walls of *Datura innoxia* Suspension Cell Cultures." *In Vitro Cellular and Developmental Biology-Plant* 29 (1994): 220–26.
4. W. F. Mueller, G. W. Bedell, S. Shojaee, and P. J. Jackson, "Bioremediation of TNT Wastes by Higher Plants," in *Proceedings of the 10th Annual Conference on Hazardous Waste Research* (Los Alamos: New Mexico State University, 1995).

RED CLOVER

1. William Shakespeare, *Titus Andronicus* (New York: Simon & Schuster, 2005), act 4, scene 4, line 90.

ROSEMARY

1. W. R. Biers and P. E. McGovern, eds., "Organic Contents of Ancient Vessels: Materials Analysis and Archaeological Investigation," *MASCA Research Papers in Science and Archaeology* 7 (1990): 25–36.

SELF-HEAL

1. Andrew Lang, *The Grey Fairy Book* (1900; repr., Mineola, N.Y.: Dover Publications, 1967).
2. Margaret Grieve, *A Modern Herbal* (Mineola, N.Y.: Dover Publications, 1971), 732.
3 Ralph Waldo Emerson, "Fortune of the Republic" (lecture delivered at the Old South Church, March 30, 1878).

SWEET BASIL

1. J. Gertsch, M. Leonti, S. Raduner, I. Racz, Jian-Zhong Chen, Xiang-Qun Xie, Karl-Heinz Altmann, M. Karsak, and A. Zimmer, "Beta-Caryophyllene Is a Dietary Cannabinoid," *Proceedings of the National Academy of Sciences of the United States of America* 105, no. 26 (2008): 9099–104.
2. Andrew Gregorovich, "Christmas Traditions of Ukraine," *Forum: A Ukrainian Review* 52 (Fall 1982): 34.

UVA URSI

1. Cedric F. Garland, Sharif B. Mohr, Frank C. Garland, Edward D. Gorham, and William B. Grant, "Lack of Sunlight Linked to Bladder Cancer," *American Journal of Preventive Medicine* (March 2010), 296–302.
2. Saikat Chatterjee, "Fair-Skin Fashion Boosts Sales of Whitening Creams in India," *Bloomberg,* November 12, 2009, www.bloomberg.com/apps/news?pid=newsarchive&sid=a.FojzJYZC.g.

Bibliography

Anderson, Michelle D. *"Ephedra viridis."* In *Fire Effects Information System.* U.S. Department of Agriculture, Forest Service, Rocky Mountain Research Station, Fire Sciences Laboratory, 2001. Available at www.fs.fed.us/database/feis (accessed December 12, 2010).

Avery, A., G. Amos, S. Satina, and J. Rietsema, *Blakeslee: The Genus* Datura. New York: Ronald Press, 1959.

Bakhru, H. K. *Herbs That Heal: Natural Remedies for Good Health.* New Delhi, India: Orient Paperbacks, 1990.

Ball, Ann. *Catholic Traditions in the Garden.* Huntington, Ind.: Our Sunday Visitor Publishing, 1998.

Bang, Seo-Hyun, Sang-Jun Han, and Dong-Hyun Kim. "Hydrolysis of Arbutin to Hydroquinone by Human Skin Bacteria and Its Effect on Antioxidant Activity." *Journal of Cosmetic Dermatology* 7, no. 3 (2010): 189–93.

Barrett, Patricia R. *Growing & Using Lavender.* Storey's Country Wisdom Bulletin A-155. North Adams, Mass.: Storey Publishing, 1996.

Beyerl, Paul. *A Compendium of Herbal Magick.* Blaine, Wash.: Phoenix Publishing, 1998.

Bicchi, C., P. Rubiolo, H. Marschall, P. Weyerstahl, and R. Laurent. "Constituents of *Artemisia roxburghiana besser* Essential Oil." *Flavor and Fragrance Journal* 13 (1998): 40–46.

Borek, Theodore T., James M. Hochrein, and Adriane N. Irwin. *Composition of the Essential Oils from Rocky Mountain Juniper* (Juniperus scopulorum), *Big Sagebrush* (Artemisia tridentata), *and White Sage* (Salvia apiana). Sandia Report SAND2003-3081. Albuquerque, N. Mex. and Livermore, Calif.: Sandia National Laboratories, 2003.

Bowers, Janice. *Shrubs and Trees of the Southwest Deserts.* Tucson, Ariz.: Western National Parks Association, 1993.

Braden, Gregg S. *Awakening to Zero Point: The Collective Initiation.* Taos, N. Mex.: Sacred Spaces Ancient Wisdom, 1994.

———. *Walking Between the Worlds: The Science of Compassion.* Taos, N. Mex.: Sacred Spaces Ancient Wisdom, 1997.

Buhner, Stephen Harrod. *The Lost Language of Plants.* White River Junction, Vt.: Chelsea Green, 2002.

Chiej, R. *The MacDonald Encyclopedia of Medicinal Plants.* London: MacDonald & Co., 1984.

Corvin-Blackburn, Judith. *Journey to Wholeness: A Guide to Inner Healing.* Springfield, Ill.: Healing Concepts Publishing, 1996.

Cowan, Eliot. *Plant Spirit Medicine.* Columbus, N.C.: Swan Raven & Co., 1995.

Darrah, Helen H. *The Cultivated Basils.* Independence, Mo.: Buckeye, 1980.

Dittberner, Phillip L., and Michael R. Olson. *The Plant Information Network (PIN) Data Base: Colorado, Montana, North Dakota, Utah, and Wyoming.* FWS/OBS-83/86. Washington, D.C.: U.S. Department of the Interior, Fish and Wildlife Service, 1983.

Duke, James A., and Steven Foster. "Eastern Central Medicinal Plants and Herbs." In *Peterson Field Guide.* Boston: Houghton Mifflin Harcourt, 1999.

Dunmire, W. W., and G. D. Tierney. *Wild Plants of the Pueblo Province.* Santa Fe: New Mexico Press, 1991.

Elpel, Thomas J. *Botany in a Day: The Patterns Method of Plant Identification.* Silver Star, Mont.: HOPS Press, 2004.

Ensminger, Audrey H., M. K. Esminger, J. E. Konlande, and J. R. K Robson. *Food for Health: A Nutrition Encyclopedia.* Clovis, Calif.: Pegus Press, 1986.

Estes, Clarissa Pinkola. *Women Who Run with the Wolves.* New York: Ballantine Books, 1996.

European Commission of Health and Consumer Protection Directorate-General. *Opinion of the Scientific Committee on Food on Thujone.* Brussels, Belgium: European Commission of Health and Consumer Protection Directorate-General, 2003.

Facciola, Stephen. *Cornucopia: A Source Book of Edible Plants.* Vista, Calif.: Kampong, 1990.

Fang, X., R. C. Chang, W. H. Yuen, and S. Y. Zee. "Immune Modulatory Effects of *Prunella Vulgaris L.*" *International Journal of Molecular Medicine* 15, no. 3 (March 2005): 491–96.

Fire, John, and Richard Erdoes. *Lame Deer, Seeker of Visions*. New York: Pocket Books, 1976.

Fox, Matthew. *The Hidden Spirituality of Men*. Novato, Calif.: New World Library, 2008.

Garrett, J. T. *The Cherokee Herbal*. Rochester, Vt.: Bear & Company, 2003.

Glenn, Evelyn Nakano. *Shades of Difference: Why Skin Color Matters*. Palo Alto, Calif.: Stanford University Press, 2009: 177–88.

Green, Mindy. *Calendula*. New York: McGraw-Hill, 1999.

Grieve, Margaret. *A Modern Herbal*. New York: Harcourt, Brace & Company, 1931. Reprint, Mineola, N.Y.: Dover, 1971.

Harner, Michael J. *The Jívaro: People of the Sacred Waterfalls*. Berkeley: University of California Press, 1984.

Harper, Douglas. *Online Etymology Dictionary*. 2001–2010. Available at www.etymonline.com.

Hatler, David F. "Food Habits of Black Bears in Interior Alaska." *Canadian Field-Naturalist* 86, no. 1 (1972): 17–31.

Hawken, Paul. *Magic of Findhorn*. New York: Bantam Books, 1975.

Hoffman, David. *Medical Herbalism: The Science and Practice of Herbal Medicine*. Rochester, Vt.: Healing Arts Press, 2003.

Hunter, Robert, John Alfred Williams, and Sidney John Hervon Herrtage. *American Encyclopedic Dictionary*. New York: Peale and J. A. Hill, 1897. This is a Google e-book. Please go to http://books.google.com and search on "American encyclopedic dictionary."

Hutchins, Alma R. *Indian Hebology of North America*. Boston: Shambhala, 1991.

Huxley, Anthony, and Mark Griffiths. *The New RHS Dictionary of Gardening*. New York: MacMillan Press, 1992.

Kaminsky, Patricia, and Richard Katz. *Flower Essence Repertory*: *A Comprehensive Guide to North American and English Flower Essences for Emotional and Spiritual Well-Being*. Nevada City, Calif.: Flower Essence Society, 1994.

Kowalchik, Claire, and William H. Hylton, eds. *Rodale's Illustrated Encyclopedia of Herbs*. New York: Rodale, 1987.

Kuhn, M. A., and D. Winston. *Herbal Therapy and Supplements*. Philadelphia: Lippincott, 2008.

Lagasse, P., L. Goldman, A. Hobson, and Susan R. Norton, eds. *The Columbia Encyclopedia*. Sixth edition. New York: Gale Group, 2000.

Lang, Andrew. *The Grey Fairy Book*. 1900. Reprint, Mineola, N.Y.: Dover, 1967.

Larson, Jennifer. *Greek Nymphs: Myths, Cult, Lore.* New York: Oxford University Press, 2001.

Libster, Martha. *Delmar's Integrative Herb Guide for Nurses.* Florence, Ky.: Delmar Cengage Learning, 2001.

Lipton, Bruce. *The Biology of Belief.* New York: Hay House, 2008.

Lis-Balchin, Maria. *Lavender: The Genus* Lavandula *(Medicinal and Aromatic Plants—Industrial Profiles).* New York: Taylor and Francis, 2002.

Maeda, K., and M. Fukuda. "Arbutin: Mechanism of Its Depigmenting Action in Human Melanocyte Culture." *The Journal of Pharmacology and Experimental Therapeutics* (February 1996): 765–69.

Manniche, Lise. *An Ancient Egyptian Herbal.* Second edition. London: British Museum Press, 2006.

Marciniak, Barbara. *Family of Light.* Rochester, Vt.: Bear & Company, 1998.

Martin, D., J. Valdez, J. Boren, and M. Mayersohn. "Dermal Absorption of Camphor, Menthol, and Methyl Salicylate in Humans." *Journal of Clinical Pharmacology* 44, no. 10 (October 2004): 1151–57.

McKenna, Terence. *Food of the Gods: The Search for the Original Tree of Knowledge.* New York: Bantam Books, 1992.

Mehl-Madrona, Lewis. *Narrative Medicine: The Use of History and Story in the Healing Process.* Rochester, Vt.: Bear & Company, 2007.

Montgomery, Pam. *Plant Spirit Healing: A Guide to Working with Plant Consciousness.* Rochester, Vt.: Bear & Company, 2008.

Moore, Michael. *Medicinal Plants of the Mountain West.* Santa Fe: The Museum of the New Mexico Press, 1979.

Mountrose, Phillip, and Jane Mountrose. *Getting Thru to Your Soul: The Four Keys to Living Your Divine Purpose.* Arroyo Grande, Calif.: Holistic Communications, 2000.

Myss, Caroline. *Defy Gravity: Healing Beyond the Bounds of Reason.* New York: Hay House, 2009.

Nunn, J. F. *Ancient Egyptian Medicine.* Norman: University of Oklahoma Press, 1996.

Peterson, Vicki. *The Natural Food Catalogue.* London: MacDonald and Jane's, 1978.

Pink, Daniel H. *A Whole New Mind: Why Right-Brainers Will Rule the Future.* New York: Riverhead Trade, 2005.

Remphrey, W. R., T. A. Steeves, and B. R. Neal. "*Arctostaphylos Uva-Ursi* (Bearberry):

An Architectural Analysis." *Canadian Journal of Botany* 61 (1983): 2430–50.

Renfrew, Colin. *Prehistory: The Making of the Human Mind.* New York: Modern Library, 2008.

Sams, Jamie, and David Carson. *Medicine Cards: The Discovery of Power through the Ways of Animals.* New York: St. Martin's Press, 1999.

Savinelli, Alfred. *Plants of Power.* Taos, N. Mex.: Native Scents, 1997.

Scully, Nicki, and Linda Star Wolf. *Shamanic Mysteries of Egypt.* Rochester, Vt.: Bear & Company, 2007.

Shlain, Leonard. *Art and Physics: Parallel Visions in Space, Time and Light.* New York: Perennial, Harper Collins, 1993.

Smith, William, ed. *Dictionary of Greek and Roman Biography and Mythology.* New York: Little and Brown, 1849.

Star Wolf, Linda, and Ruby Falconer. *Shamanic Egyptian Astrology: Your Planetary Relationship to the Gods.* Rochester, Vt.: Bear & Company, 2010.

Stearn, William T. *Botanical Latin.* Fourth edition. Portland, Ore.: Timber Press, 2004.

Stiles, Edmund W. "Patterns of Fruit Presentation and Seed Dispersal in Bird-Disseminated Woody Plants in the Eastern Deciduous Forest." *American Naturalist* 116, no. 5 (1980): 670–88.

Tedlock, Barbara. *The Woman in the Shaman's Body.* New York: Bantam Books, 2005.

Three Initiates. *The Kybalion: A Study of Hermetic Philosophy of Ancient Egypt and Greece.* Chicago: Yogi Publication Society, Masonic Temple, 1912, 1940.

Tisserand, R., and T. Balacs. *Essential Oil Safety.* Edinburgh, Scotland: Churchill-Livingstone, 1995.

Tschense, Nicholas. "Bringer of Light and Love." Available at www.nicholastschense.com/Poetry_Indigo_Children.html.

Upson, Tim, and Susyn Andrews. *The Genus* Lavandula. Portland, Ore.: Timber Press, 2004.

Vaughan, Frances E. *Awakening Intuition.* New York: Anchor Books, 1978.

Waters, Frank. *Book of the Hopi.* New York: Penguin, 1963.

Watson-Kamm, Minnie. *Old Time Herbs for Northern Gardeners.* New York: Dover, 1971.

Weed, Susun. *Healing Wise.* Woodstock, N.Y.: Ash Tree, 1989.

———. *Menopausal Years: The Wise Woman Way.* Woodstock, N.Y.: Ash Tree, 1992.

Wichtl, M., ed. *Herbal Drugs and Phytopharmaceuticals.* Translated by Josef A. Brinckmann and Michael P. Lindenmaier. Third edition. Stuttgart, Germany: Medpharm Scientific Publishers, 2004.

Wilkinson, T. J., and P. Murphy. "Archaeological Survey of an Intertidal Zone: The Submerged Landscape of the Essex Coast, England." *Journal of Field Archaeology* 13, no. 2 (Summer 1986): 177–94.

Wright, Machaelle Small. *Behaving as if the God in All Life Mattered.* Warrenton, Va.: Perelandra, 1997.

Yarnell, Eric. "Misunderstood 'Toxic' Herbs." *Alternative & Complementary Therapies* (February 1999): 6–11.

About the Author

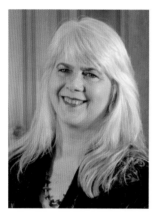

Thea Summer Deer is an award-winning singer-songwriter, licensed minister (through Madonna Ministries: a global spiritual community), and a Shamanic High Priestess (Priestess Process). She has been a student of metaphysics and the healing arts for more than thirty-five years, having been educated by herbalists across the United States, Canada, and Europe. She is currently studying for her doctorate through Venus Rising University in Whittier, North Carolina. Thea was the executive director of Resources for World Health, located in San Francisco, a non-profit research organization that supports indigenous healers within their communities. She owned and operated the Mindbody and Evolutionary Press, also in San Francisco, in partnership with Lewis Mehl-Madrona, M.D., Ph.D. She has been a pipe carrier, leader of sweat lodges, and presenter of workshops on the shamanic healing arts. Thea is currently a shamanic minister, clinical herbalist, and educator. Her website is www.theasummerdeer.com.

Index

Page numbers in *italics* refer to illustrations.

survival, 159

sweet basil, 164–73, *164*

  deva speaks, 171–73

  divination of, 169–71

  effects of, 167, 184, 185

  history of, 165–66

  sovereignty and, 169–73

  uses of, 167–69

Sweet King, 171–72

sympathetic resonance, 15

Symphytum officinale. See comfrey

synergy, 3

tarragon, 135

teas, 1–2

technology, 143

Theosophical Society, 11

third eye, 12

thought, 15

threshold effects, 148

time, 16, 141–43, 146–48

Time Keepers, 141–46

time travel, 145–46

tinctures, 1–2

tobacco, 176

tonics, 1–2

Trifolium pratense. See red clover

trinity, 122

truth, 41

tulsi, 166

Tyler, Varro, 59

unconditional love, 157–62

unification theory, 16

unity, 94

urinary tract infections, 177, 179–80

Ute, 139

uva ursi, 174–83, *174*

  description of, 175–76

  deva speaks, 180–83

  divination of, 179–80

  effects of, 184

  history of, 175–76

  introspection and, 179–83

  uses of, 177–78

Venus, 17, 170

vibrational medicine, 6

Virgin Mary, 128

Vishnu, 36

Vogel, Marcel, 15, 38

vulgaris, 153–54

Weed, Susun, 3

weeds, 157, 163

White Buffalo Calf Woman, 170

wholeness, 62–65

wildlife, 138, 176–77

wisdom, 2

Wise Woman Tradition, 3

wormwood, 135

Wright, Charles, 70

Wright, Machaelle Small, 3

yielding, 27

yoga, 12

BOOKS OF RELATED INTEREST

The Secret Teachings of Plants
The Intelligence of the Heart in the Direct Perception of Nature
by Stephen Harrod Buhner

Sacred Plant Medicine
The Wisdom in Native American Herbalism
by Stephen Harrod Buhner

Plant Spirit Healing
A Guide to Working with Plant Consciousness
by Pam Montgomery

Ecomysticism
The Profound Experience of Nature as Spiritual Guide
by Carl von Essen, M.D.

Plant Spirit Shamanism
Traditional Techniques for Healing the Soul
by Ross Heaven and Howard G. Charing

Planetary Healing
Spirit Medicine for Global Transformation
by Nicki Scully and Mark Hallert

The Cherokee Herbal
Native Plant Medicine from the Four Directions
by J. T. Garrett

Coyote Healing
Miracles in Native Medicine
by Lewis Mehl-Madrona, M.D., Ph.D.

INNER TRADITIONS • BEAR & COMPANY
P.O. Box 388
Rochester, VT 05767
1-800-246-8648
www.InnerTraditions.com

Or contact your local bookseller